A HANDBOOK OF OBSTETRIC AND GYNECOLOGIC EMERGENCIES

A HANDBOOK OF OBSTETRIC AND GYNECOLOGIC EMERGENCIES

Editors

S. ARULKUMARAN

MD, PhD, FRCS, FRCOG, FACOG, FAMS
Professor and Head, Department of Obstetrics and Gynecology
St. George's Hospital Medical College, London

K.BHASKER RAO

MD, FRCOG, FAMS
Senior Consultant Obstetrician and Gynecologist
Vijaya Hospital, Chennai
Former Director
Institute of Obstetrics and Gynecology, Chennai

MALA VIJAYAKRISHNAN

MD, DGO,
Senior Consultant Obstetrician and Gynecologist
Vijaya Hospital, Chennai

Orient Longman

Orient Longman Private Limited

Registered Office

3-6-752 Himayatnagar, Hyderabad 500 029 (A.P.) India

Other Offices

Bangalore/Bhopal/Bhubaneshwar/Chennai/
Ernakulam/Guwahati/Hyderabad/Jaipur/Kolkata/
Lucknow/Mumbai/New Delhi/Patna

First published 2003

ISBN 81 250 2516 2

Typeset by

Trinity Designers & Typesetters
Chennai 600 041

Printed in India by offset at

Novena Offset Print Co
Chennai 600 005

Published by

Orient Longman Private Limited
160 Anna Salai
Chennai 600 002

Preface

Maternal mortality and temporary or permanent morbidity following pregnancy and childbirth are a reality for millions of women. Of the 600,000 women who die each year of childbirth and related conditions, 99 per cent are from the developing world, mainly from Africa and Southeast Asia (particularly India). The vast majority of women do not (and often cannot) avail of antenatal care or afford a childbirth attended by a professionally trained person. Many childbirths take place outside hospital settings. Fortunately, the vast majority of pregnancies and childbirth are normal.

When pregnancy becomes high-risk or abnormal, it becomes an emergency, and without adequate care the mother and child succumb to the condition or suffer the consequences (general disability or reproductive ill health). Many women seek refuge in primary healthcare centres or hospitals, where inadequate obstetric care and facilities are available. The physicians and paramedics should be able to anticipate these emergencies, detect them early and treat them promptly, if we are to see improvement in mortality and morbidity. This handbook *Obstetric and Gynecologic Emergencies* is written with this intent in mind. It is a pocket book to be used by the physician or administrator in the clinic or health setting. It spells out the presentation, clinical features to help in diagnosis, differential diagnosis and management. It gives specific advice about what to do in such emergencies, rather than state what others do.

In a healthcare setting, the physician or paramedic attends to emergencies other than of obstetrics and gynecology. This text is not exhaustive and is only tailored to cover obstetric and gynecologic emergencies. Many conditions and emergencies are described, but it may not be possible to manage every condition within a given setting. This handbook provides advice on prevention and also the appropriate facilities that should be available to manage a specific condition. It also lists out the initial steps that should be taken prior to appropriate referral. The editors are conscious of the three delay model, delay in seeking treatment; delay in reaching a healthcare facility; and delay in obtaining definitive treatment in the facility. If the physician does not have adequate knowledge of the condition, the third kind of delay is prolonged even more; as a consequence morbidity and mortality increase. We have kept this in mind when producing this book and sincerely hope it will be useful to administrators, physicians and paramedical staff.

S. Arulkumaran
K. Bhasker Rao
Mala Vijayakrishnan

Acknowledgement

The editors and publishers are grateful to the World Health Organization for permission to reproduce the following figures from *Managing Complications in Pregnancy and Childbirth: A Guide for Midwives and Doctors*, 2000. Figures P2, P5, P6, P8, P9, P10, P11, P12, P14, P15, P17, P20, P21, P24, P28, P30, P31, P38, P42, P43, P45, P52, P55, P57, S26, S27.

Contents

Contributors

1. **S. Arulkumaran,** MD, PhD, FRCS, FRCOG, FACOG, FAMS
Professor and Head of Department
St. George's Hospital Medical College
London

2. **S. Jayam,** MD, DCh
Senior Consultant Pediatrician
Vijaya Health Centre, Chennai
Formerly Director
Institute of Child Health, Chennai

3. **Dilip Karnad,** MD, MNAMS
Consultant Critical Care
KEM Hospital, Mumbai

4. **Kumari Menon,** MBBS, DCh
Consultant Neonatologist
Vijaya Hospital, Chennai

5. **Surajit Mitra,** MD, MRCOG
Associate Specialist
Department of Obstetrics and Gynecology
Medical School, Nottingham
United Kingdom

6. **Mona Pandurangi,** MD
Consultant Gynecologist
Vijaya Hospital, Chennai

7. **K. Bhasker Rao,** MD, FRCOG, FAMS
Senior Consultant Obstetrician and Gynecologist
Vijaya Hospital, Chennai
Former Director
Institute of Obstetrics and Gynecology, Chennai

8. **Mala Vijayakrishnan,** MD, DGO
Senior Consultant Obstetrician and Gynecologist
Vijaya Hospital, Chennai

9. **B V Reddy,** MD, DA
Consultant Anesthesiologist
Vijaya Hospital, Chennai

Abbreviations

ACE	Angiotensin converting enzyme
AMI	Acute myocardial infarction
APH	Antepartum hemorrhage
ARM	Artificial rupture of membranes
BD	Twice daily
BOH	Bad obstetric history
BP	Blood pressure
CPD	Cephalopelvic disproportion
CS	Cesarean section
CTG	Cardiotocography
CX	Cervix
DBP	Diastolic blood pressure
DHEA	Dihydroepiandrosterone
DMPA	Depot medroxy progesterone acetate
DUB	Dysfunctional uterine bleeding
ECV	External cephalic version
EDD	Expected date of delivery
FFN	Fetal fibronectin
FH	Fetal heart
FHR	Fetal heart rate
HB	Hemoglobin
HBI_g	Hepatitis B immunoglobulin
HCG	Human chorionic gonadotropin
HCT	Hematocrit
HDP	Hypertensive diseases of pregnancy
HELLP	Hemolysis, elevated liver enzymes, low platelet counts
ICV	Internal cephalic version

IHCP	Intrahepatic cholestosis of pregnancy
IM	Intramuscular
IUCD	Intrauterine copper releasing device
IUD	Intrauterine death
IUGR	Intrauterine growth restriction
IV	Intravenous
IVF	In vitro fertilisation
LBW	Low birth weight
LOA	Left occipito anterior
L/S	Lecithin sphingomyelin
$MgSO_4$	Magnesium sulphate
NMR	Neonatal mortality rate
NST	Non-stress test
PG	Prostaglandin
PGE_2	Prostaglandin E_2
PGF_{2a}	Prostaglandin $F_2 \alpha$
PID	Pelvic inflammatory disease
PIH	Pregnancy induced hypertension
PMR	Perinatal mortality rate
PPH	Post partum hemorrhage
PPROM	Preterm prelabour rupture of membranes
PROM	Prelabour rupture of membranes
PV	Per vaginum
QD	Four times daily
QID	Once daily
ROP	Right occipito posterior
ROT	Right occipito transverse
SGA	Small for gestational age
SLE	Systemic lupus erythematosus
SVD	Spontaneous vaginal delivery
TID	Thrice daily
USG	Ultrasonograph[y]

1. Introduction

Of an estimated half a million mothers who die annually worldwide, due to complications of pregnancy and labour, 99 per cent are from developing countries. India alone contributes to 25 per cent of these maternal deaths due to its large population, poor maternity care and high maternal mortality rate (MMR) of 437 per 100,000 births, compared to 30 in Sri Lanka, 10 in Singapore and 6 in Norway.

Reports from the developing world have shown that about 80 per cent of all maternal deaths are due to direct obstetric causes and 20 per cent are due to indirect causes (such as anemia, malaria and viral hepatitis complicating pregnancy). Among the direct causes, hemorrhages of pregnancy, especially postpartum hemorrhage (PPH), are the commonest, followed by sepsis, eclampsia, obstructed labour and unsafe abortions. Most of these complications can be prevented, or detected early. Prompt treatment can save these mothers.

An emergency may be defined as an unexpected occurrence requiring immediate attention. Any delay in such situations entails grave consequences. About 15 per cent of all women may report with an emergency during pregnancy, labour and puerperium. In obstetrics, if an emergency is not properly treated it may endanger the life or health of not only the mother, but also her child. In gynecological emergencies delay may not only pose a threat to the life of the woman, but also affect her chances of reproduction. *Pregnancy is a period of (usually low) risk. However, the risk may be enhanced when the pregnancy is associated with certain factors or when it is unsupervised. It is not possible to predict which mother may develop complications before or during delivery.* In one study, 25 per cent of nulliparas and 10 per cent of multiparas in the 'low-risk' group had unforeseen emergencies in labour.

In large cities, even in developing countries, there are well-equipped and well-staffed maternity institutions. Transport too is readily available so that these emergencies are generally attended to with minimum delay. However, most deliveries and obstetric emergencies occur in rural areas where health care facilities are poor and rapid transportation services are scarce. Even after finally reaching a referral hospital (usually a district/sub-district hospital) after several hours, there is often a further delay of 2 to 3 hours before necessary intervention is initiated.

The World Health Organization therefore recommends, that to reduce maternal deaths, these obstetric complications or emergencies should be treated at a first referral level closer to the patient's home, by physicians specially trained in emergency obstetric care and who can carry out essential obstetric functions. The first referral centre may be defined as the most peripheral hospital at which adequate care for obstetric emergencies is available.

The essential obstetric functions are:

1. Surgical functions: Ability to perform laparotomy, cesarean section, ectopic gestation, repair of ruptured uterus or cervical tear, amniotomy/oxytocin drip, evacuation of the uterus in an abortion.
2. Anesthetic functions: To administer general, regional or local anesthesia
3. Medical treatment functions: Management of shock/ hemorrhage, sepsis, anemia, severe pregnancy induced hypertension (PIH) including eclampsia.
4. Blood replacement: Typing, cross-matching, and transfusion for surgery, hemorrhages or severe anemia
5. Manual functions: Partography, vacuum extraction or outlet forceps delivery, manual removal of the placenta

6. Management of high-risk cases: Identification, referral and treatment of high-risk pregnant women. High-risk women may be identified from:
   - Previous history (of stillbirth, neonatal death, low birth weight (LBW), macrosomia, and repeated abortions), treatment of high blood pressure, cesarean section and PPH
   - Present pregnancy (age under 16 years or over 35 years, twins, Rh factor, vaginal bleeding and PIH)
   - Associated medical conditions like anemia, heart disease, jaundice
7. Family planning functions: Male and female sterilisation, oral pills and intrauterine device (IUD) insertions.
8. Neonatal care: Neonatal resuscitation, prevention of hypothermia and early breast-feeding

It is essential for safe motherhood that there should be close co-operation between the community, field staff and the hospital staff, as well as the availability of rapid transportation, communication and blood transfusion services.

When faced with an emergency the team leader should mobilise the team quickly. The team should also practise an emergency drill at short notice to treat cases of eclampsia, hemorrhage and arrested labour so that the staff is always alert and ready to tackle emergencies. In an emergency situation the hospital staff should also have good communication skills. At the time of admission, the patient and her immediate family must be informed about her present condition, type of management proposed and the likely outcome. In case of stillbirth or neonatal death, circumstances surrounding the tragedy should be explained, including future prospects.

Primary maternal health care is extremely important and in developing countries it should be prioritised if the maternal mortality/morbidity rate is to be low. The delivery of maternity care at this level should include:

1. Registration, examination and advice in early pregnancy, before twelve weeks and subsequent three visits (around 26 weeks, 32 weeks, and 38 weeks) before the delivery.

She should be immunised against tetanus and be given iron and folic acid orally to prevent/treat anemia. At each visit careful monitoring of the mother and the fetus is carried out. At the last visit a decision is made as to the place of delivery. By reducing the number of prenatal visits to four, no difference in the maternal or fetal outcome was noticed in a large multicentric study.

2. A trained attendant should supervise each birth.
3. Referral facilities for high-risk pregnancies and obstetric emergencies should be available.
4. Postnatally, universal breast-feeding, immunisation of infants and acceptance of family planning by mothers should be encouraged.

Though several textbooks in obstetrics and gynecology are available, when faced with an emergency a practical guide or a manual is extremely useful to quickly arrive at a diagnosis and plan appropriate treatment. This manual deals with obstetric and gynecological emergencies commonly encountered in community practice. Typical case reports are given as examples so that one can easily arrive at a diagnosis, rapidly assess the case at hand and decide on the appropriate therapeutic steps. The prognosis and the likely complications one might encounter during emergencies are also given, as well as ways of coping with these. Preventive measures are included so that these emergencies can be prevented where possible.

This handbook is meant for physicians working in peripheral areas at the first referral centres and for residents undergoing training in obstetrics and gynecology. It will also be useful for general practitioners who may come across such emergencies in their practice. A list of references at the end of each chapter is only to help further reading and does not cover the subject comprehensively.

It is important to realise that there are limitations to what could be done at these centres and on deciding what type of cases need referral to tertiary care level hospitals. However, in this book the options are deliberately restricted to procedures that could be carried out by a physician with limited experience in anesthesia, obstetrics or surgery using facilities that are usually expected at such first referral centres.

The editors hope that this manual will contribute to the prevention of maternal mortality, promotion of maternal health, and advancement of emergency skills in developing countries.

Bibliography

World Health Organization 1996. The global coverage of maternity care. 4th edn Geneva: WHO.

UNFPA 1999. *State of the world's population*. New York: UNFPA, p 68

Berglund A and Lindmark G 2000. Risk assessment at the end of pregnancy. *Acta Obstet Gynecol Scand* 79: 854-859.

World Health Organization 1996. The essential obstetric functions at first referral level. Report of a technical working group. Geneva: WHO.

Villar J, Ba'qeel H, Piaggio G et al 2001. WHO antenatal care randomized trial for the evaluation of a new model of routine antenatal care. *Lancet* 357: 1551–64.

World Health Organization 1999. Reduction of maternal mortality. Joint statement of WHO, UNFPA, UNICEF. Geneva: WHO, p 20.

2. Bleeding in early pregnancy

Any bleeding in the early weeks of pregnancy (before 22 weeks) may be due to:

- Abortion
- Hydatidiform mole
- Ectopic gestation
- Associated lesions (cervical polyps and carcinoma)

ABORTION

Abortion is defined as termination of pregnancy prior to 22 weeks or before the viability of the fetus, or when the conceptus weighs 500 g or less.

Incidence

It may be spontaneous in 15 per cent of pregnancies.

Types

It may be spontaneous or induced. Induced abortions may be therapeutic (legal) or unsafe (see pp 10-11). Unsafe abortions are those performed by untrained persons in unhygienic conditions.

SPONTANEOUS ABORTION

Etiology

Over 60 per cent of early abortions are due to chromosomal anomalies in the conceptus (aneuploidy, autosomal trisomy and polyploidy, in order of frequency). In early habitual abortions, chromosomal translocations have to be ruled out by studying the maternal and paternal chromosomes from peripheral blood. In mid-trimester abortions the causes to be considered are congenital uterine anomalies, cervical incompetence, endocrine (thyroid) or metabolic disorder (diabetes) and thrombophilia. Though periconceptional folic acid helps prevent neural tube defects, its supplementation before or during pregnancy does not decrease chances of miscarriage.

Types and diagnosis

Spontaneous abortion (also called miscarriage) may be of several types (Fig 2.1). Ultrasonography (USG) can help distinguish between the various types of abortion.

1. *Threatened:* When there is very little pain and bleeding, the cervix is closed, and the uterus corresponds to the period of amenorrhea. In centres where ultrasound facilities are available, fetal heart action could be seen after 6 weeks. There is a possibility of continuation of pregnancy with rest and treatment
2. *Inevitable:* When the pain and bleeding increases. The cervical os is usually open and the conceptus is felt.
3. *Incomplete:* When part of the conceptus is expelled. The cervix is usually open and the uterus is small for the gestation period.
4. *Complete:* When the uterus is empty. The cervix may be closed and the uterus is small for the gestation period.
5. *Missed:* After its death the embryo or the fetus is retained in the uterus. In such a case the cervix is closed and uterine size is small for the period of amenorrhea. The pregnancy test will be positive for some time and may take upto 5 to 6 weeks to be negative, as the trophoblastic tissue continues to secrete β-hCG, detection of which forms the basis of the pregnancy test.

Treatment

In *threatened miscarriage*, the treatment is rest, with no sexual

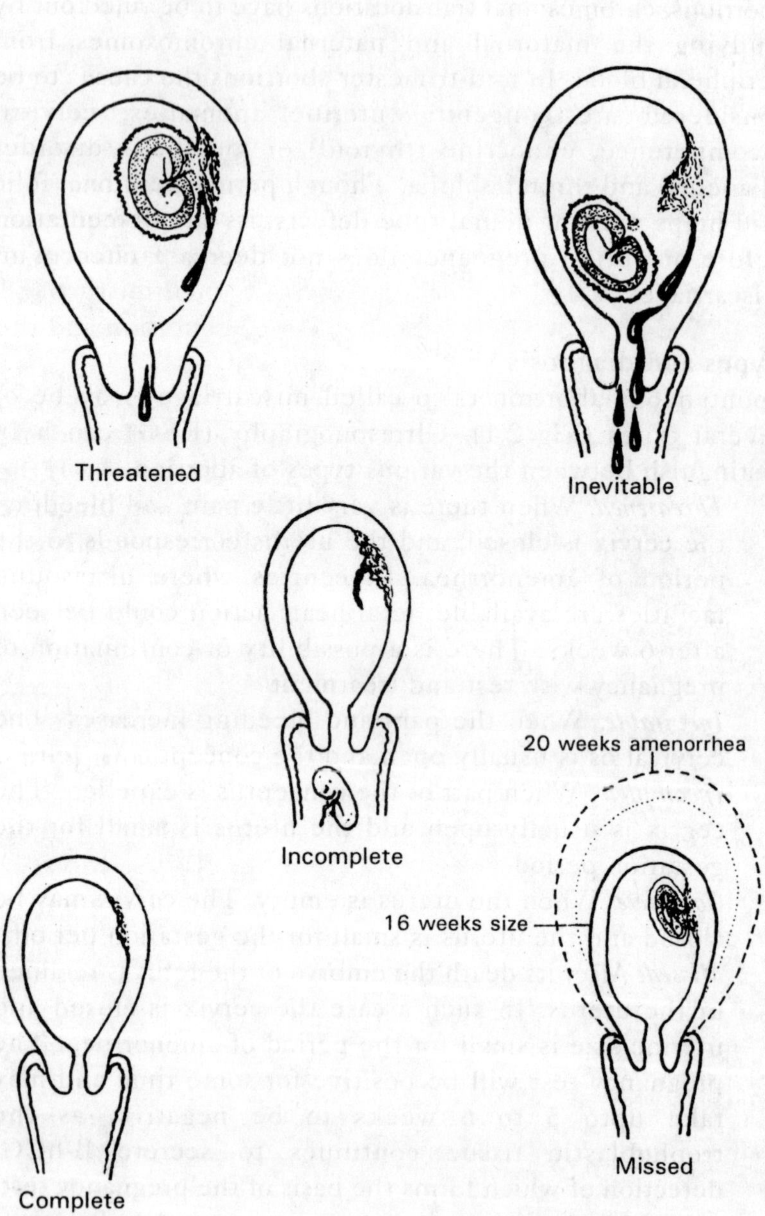

Fig 2.1 Types of spontaneous abortion

intercourse till the bleeding stops. There is no place for any hormonal or tocolytic therapy. The pregnancy test and USG could be done where facilities are available. If the USG shows the FH activity, the chances of continuing the pregnancy are about 95 per cent. The bleeding in pregnancy is associated with a 2–3 fold increase in the risk of premature birth.

In *inevitable abortion*, there is no chance of continuation of pregnancy, as the conceptus has already separated. The pain and bleeding are more than in threatened miscarriage. The management depends on the general condition and the duration of pregnancy.

- If gestation is less than 16 weeks, the cervix is open or admits a finger, and the conceptus is felt, it could be removed digitally or with a sponge-forceps. If the cervix is closed and there is very little bleeding, she is given 400 μg of misoprostol orally or vaginally and it could be repeated 6 hours later if needed.
- If the gestation is more than 16 weeks, and the uterus is palpable, oxytocin 20 units in 500 ml of normal saline is given intravenously at the rate of 20 drops per minute. Alternatively, misoprostol 400 μg can be given vaginally at three hour intervals up to a maximum of five doses.

In *incomplete abortion* of less than 16 weeks, the remaining bits of conceptus could be digitally removed if the cervix is open. If there is bleeding and the cervix does not admit a finger, vacuum aspiration and curettage is indicated. After 16 weeks, the placenta is usually retained and the oxytocin drip (as suggested earlier) is required. If there is no response, the uterus needs to be evacuated by vacuum aspiration or curettage.

Missed abortion is diagnosed from the patient's previous history and clinical findings – cessation of further growth of the uterus, negative pregnancy test (late presentation), and absence of fetal heart and fetal activity on ultrasonography. In such cases the uterus could be emptied by administration of 400 μg of misoprostol vaginally and repeated if necessary every 4 to 6 hours for 24 hours. This regimen can be repeated if necessary, preferably after 12 to 24 hours of rest.

If the pregnancy is of more than 16 weeks, it is managed as suggested in chapter 6 (pp 48) ('Absence of fetal movements').

All cases of complete miscarriage will need follow up advice:

1. About future contraception: For spacing, a copper IUCD can be introduced at the end of the procedure or prior to discharge. Alternatively, the patient is advised hormonal contraception. If she is a parous woman, tubal ligation is offered (chapter 3).
2. She may need Rh anti-D immunisation if she is Rh negative, and also tetanus immunisation if not given in the last two years.
3. She is also advised to take oral iron for the next 6 weeks.

In *septic abortions* the retained conceptus is infected by pathogenic organisms of the coliform or clostridial group. Though they are usually unsafe abortions, septic abortions may sometimes follow a spontaneous incomplete abortion.

Case Report 1

An 18-year-old unmarried girl is admitted with history of 2 months amenorrhea, lower abdominal pain, vomiting, and fever for 2 days. She denies history of any interference. On examination she looks ill, not anemic, pulse 118 per min, BP 110/70, temp 39°C. Lower abdominal tenderness and slight rigidity are present. Pelvic examination reveals slight offensive blood stained discharge. Cervix is torn on the left side, and the uterus is bulky with tenderness of the fornices but no palpable mass.

Discussion

This unmarried teenager complaining of 2 months amenorrhea, lower abdominal pain, bloody discharge per vaginum and with fever and vomiting is not a case of hydatidiform mole as the uterus is not palpable. In spite of a rapid pulse there is no anemia or shock to suggest a ruptured ectopic pregnancy. It is a case of septic induced abortion with pelvic peritonitis. The offensive vaginal discharge, torn cervix, bulky uterus with tender fornices, leucocytosis, and ultrasonography showing a bit of conceptus in the slightly enlarged uterus and some amount of free fluid in the pelvis confirm the diagnosis of a septic unsafe abortion.

Management

This person is to be treated with broad spectrum antibiotics IV (chapter 18) and parenteral fluids with Ryle's tube aspiration of the stomach. If there is no response to conservative therapy in 2–3 days, laparotomy is indicated. In case there is any perforation of the uterus, it is sutured. The peritoneal fluid, purulent or serosanguinous, is drained after collecting a sample for culture. She is also given an injection of tetanus toxoid. Most patients respond to conservative therapy. Once peritonitis has subsided she is given oral feeds and medication. After she is afebrile, the uterus is evacuated 6 hours after giving her 1 g ampicillin IV; ampicillin is continued for two more days.

Complications

Complications of unsafe abortions are:

1. Septicemia
2. Septic shock
3. Tetanus/gangrene due to Clostridium tetani and welchi
4. Pelvic abscess
5. Pelvic inflammatory disease

Prevention

Unsafe abortions can be prevented by use of contraception. If this fails, safe medical termination of pregnancy by trained personnel in the appropriate setting may be undertaken.

Mortality: Mortality in unsafe abortions is about 5 per cent but if septic shock should follow, the fatality rate goes up to 35–50 per cent. Unsafe abortions account for 15 per cent of all maternal deaths

HYDATIDIFORM MOLE (OR MOLAR PREGNANCY)

This condition is seen in early weeks of pregnancy and is characterised by

1. Marked proliferation of terminal villi giving rise to excessive production of chorionic gonadotropins.
2. Hydropic degeneration of these microscopic villi into grape-like watery cysts leading to overdistension of uterus.
3. Death and resorption of the early embryo.

It is an important cause of bleeding in early pregnancy. Passage of grape-like vesicles will clinch the diagnosis. In 5 per cent of cases it leads to choriocarcinoma.

Incidence

It is seen in about 1 in 1000 pregnancies.

Etiology

The cause is not known.

> **Case Report 2**
>
> A 23-year-old primigravida reports with history of 10 weeks amenorrhea and a short bout of vaginal bleeding 3 hours ago.
>
> On examination she is not anemic and has slight pedal edema. Her BP is 130/90, pulse 86/min, Hb 10 g per cent. The uterus is about 20 weeks size, with no internal ballottement. FH is not present. There is no bleeding. The USG shows no evidence of the fetus but presents a speckled ('snow storm') appearance and β-hCG is above 100,000 iu/l.

Differential diagnosis

The differential diagnosis is given in Fig 2.2. This is a typical case of hydatidiform mole. In this case, the diagnosis is not in doubt. The disproportionately enlarged uterus with no evidence of the fetus clinically or on ultrasonography, mild PIH in early pregnancy, and excessive gonadotropin production are the pointers.

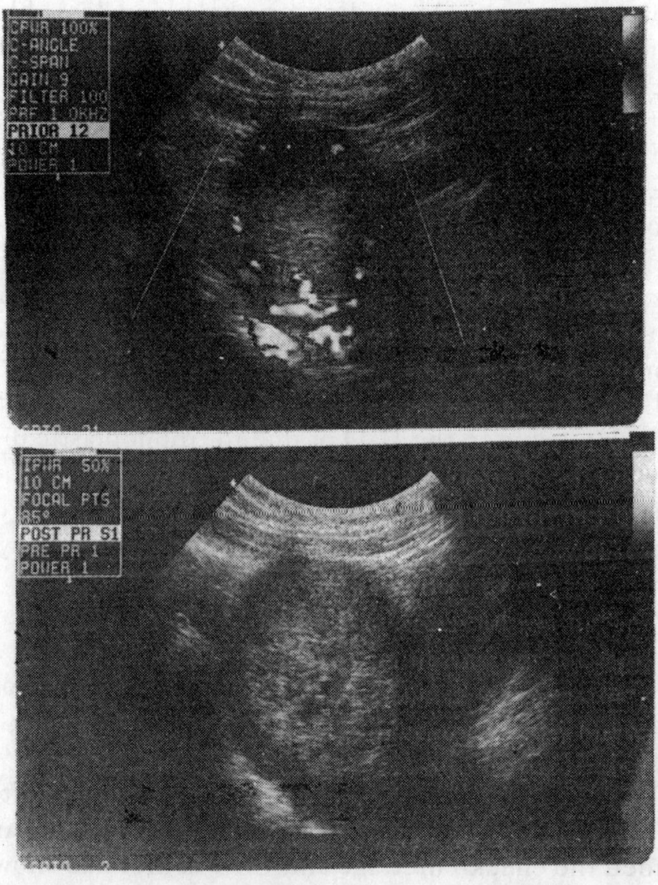

Fig 2.2 A typical ultrasonograph in case of a hydatidiform mole. The Doppler blood flow in the same case shows collection of blood in between the vesicles

Management

Once the diagnosis of hydatidiform mole is made, the uterus has to be emptied without waiting for any bleeding. Blood group and type is determined and an IV line is started with normal saline. As the cervix is closed, dilatation and vacuum aspiration with curettage is the method of choice. To prevent hemorrhage, 20 units of oxytocin is added to the saline. A check-curettage is done to ensure that the uterus is completely empty. Depending on the blood loss, blood is transfused. Ampicillin 500 mg 6 hourly is given orally to prevent infection.

Follow up

It is extremely important that all cases of hydatidiform mole are followed up clinically as well as with a hormonal assay, since the chances of developing choriocarcinoma are 1000 times more following a molar pregnancy compared to a normal pregnancy. On discharge, the patient is advised oral iron for a month, and preferably barrier contraception for a year. An IUD may produce irregular bleeding causing doubt as to whether it is due to the IUD or due to trophoblastic disease. She is seen weekly for 2 months for any bleeding. Eight weeks after the curettage the urine should be negative for a pregnancy test. Later she is advised to attend a tertiary level centre for follow up and further therapy, if necessary.

Complications and prognosis

The complications are hemorrhage, sepsis, perforation and malignancy, the risk of trophoblastic neoplasia being about 5 per cent. Careful long term follow up is essential.

When there is vaginal bleeding after a molar abortion, it may be due to either an invasive mole or choriocarcinoma, provided the check-curettage and USG earlier had shown the uterus to be empty. Hormonal assay, USG and histological examination of the curettings help the diagnosis. The major risk in an invasive mole is one of perforation with profuse intraperitoneal hemorrhage, and in choriocarcinoma of early hematogenous spread to other organs. In the prevention and treatment of gestational trophoblastic neoplasia, chemotherapy is necessary in early cases to achieve 100 per cent cure.

ECTOPIC GESTATION

Normally, the implantation of the conceptus occurs in the uterus. In ectopic gestation it occurs outside the uterus and in 95 per cent of such cases it is in the fallopian tube (Fig 2.3). As the tube is not structurally or functionally suitable to be the seat of pregnancy (because of absence of decidua and its poor musculature), tubal rupture occurs early in pregnancy leading to hemorrhagic shock. Ruptured tubal pregnancy is an acute emergency, and unless promptly treated, can be fatal (Fig 2.4).

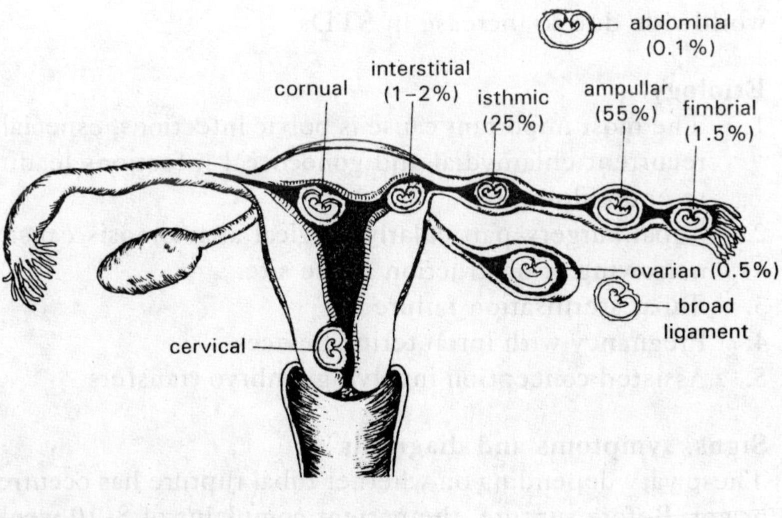

Fig 2.3 Sites of ectopic gestation. The figures in brackets show relative frequency

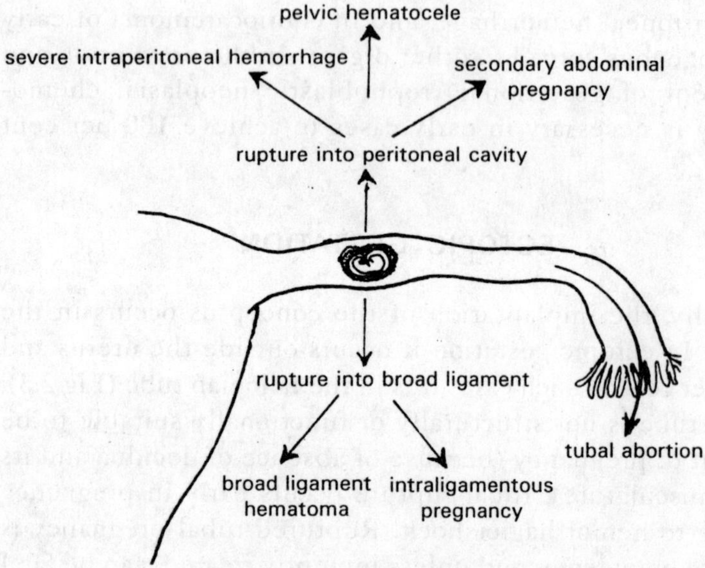

Fig 2.4 The ovum in tubal gestation

Incidence

Incidence is about 1 in 200 pregnancies, and is on the rise worldwide due to increase in STDs.

Etiology

1. The most important cause is pelvic infections, especially recurrent chlamydial and gonococcal infections leading to endosalpingitis.
2. Tubal surgery particularly surgical anastomosis causing narrowing or obstruction at the site.
3. Tubal sterilisation failure
4. Pregnancy with intrauterine devices
5. Assisted conception involving embryo transfers

Signs, symptoms and diagnosis

These vary depending on whether tubal rupture has occurred or not. Before rupture, the patient complains of 8–10 weeks amenorrhea with nausea and colicky abdominal pain. There may be slight bleeding giving the impression of a threatened miscarriage. Pregnancy test will be positive. Per vaginum, the cervix is closed and the uterus is bulky. A tender pulsatile adnexal mass may or may not be palpable. The diagnosis is made mainly on suspicion and the USG which shows an empty uterus and an adnexal mass (sometimes gestational sac with the embryo/fetus can be seen). In case of doubt, laparoscopy will confirm the diagnosis.

After rupture

After the rupture, the clinical picture is one of hemorrhagic collapse. The patient complains of lower abdominal pain, vaginal spotting or bleeding, and fainting. Examination shows pallor, rapid pulse and hypotension with lower abdominal tenderness on the side of rupture. The USG will show an empty uterus and peritoneal cavity full of blood or fluid. In most cases of acute tubal rupture there is no need for USG or diagnostic laparoscopy. The diagnosis can and should be made on clinical grounds alone. Culdocentesis (for aspiration of blood) can be done and is positive in most cases (Fig 2.5).

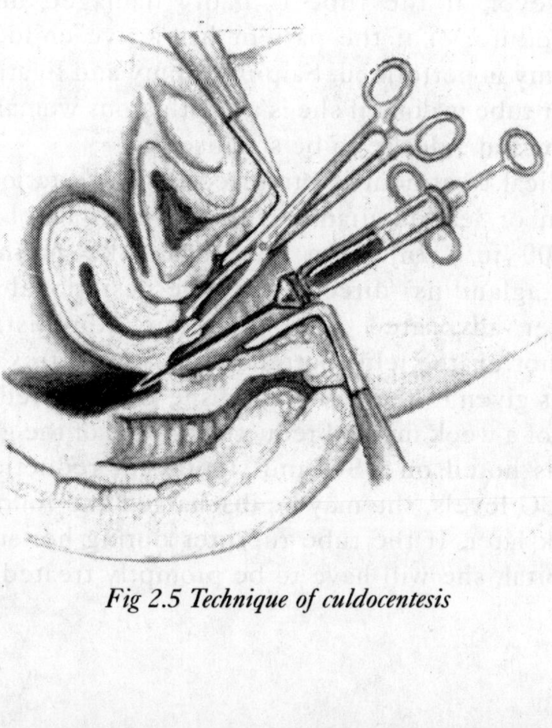

Fig 2.5 Technique of culdocentesis

Differential diagnosis: The possible differential diagnoses are (chapter 17):

1. Threatened abortion
2. Pelvic inflammatory disease (including acute salpingitis)
3. Pyelitis
4. Twisted ovarian cyst
6. Acute appendicitis

Management: Early diagnosis is extremely important for conservative medical or surgical management of tubal pregnancy and if the tube is to be salvaged.

Before rupture

1. If the gestational sac is 4 cm or more in diameter, and β-hCG level exceeds 10,000 iu/l, laparoscopic surgery is advisable. In nulliparous women, salpingostomy is the procedure of choice. A linear incision is made on the antemesenteric border of the tube, the contents are sucked out and hemostasis obtained. The pelvic cavity is flushed and the laparoscopic wound is closed. However, if the tube is badly damaged during the procedure, or if the patient has a live child, salpingectomy is performed. Salpingectomy and ligation of the other tube is done if she is a multiparous woman and had expressed a desire to be sterilised.
2. Medical treatment is preferred if the gestational sac is 3 cm or less in diameter and β-hCG level is below 10,000 iu/l. Injection of drugs (like methotrexate, prostaglandins) directly into the gestational sac is no longer advocated since systemic administration of methotrexate yields better results. Methotrexate 50 mg IM is given to the patient and she is monitored. If at the end of a week marked reduction in size of the gestational sac is noted on USG and significant reduction in the β-hCG levels, she may be discharged and followed up a week later. If the tube ruptures during her stay in the hospital, she will have to be promptly treated. Medical

treatment is not cost effective as hospitalisation is longer and there is a 15–20 per cent risk of laparotomy in case tubal rupture occurs while the patient is under observation. However, with successful medical treatment, tubal patency rates of 80 per cent are claimed with subsequent pregnancy rates of over 60 per cent. Ideally if the gestational sac was 3 cm or less and regressed with declining β-hCG values to below 1500 miu/ml, good results are obtained.

Management of ruptured ectopic pregnancy

An IV line is established with a 14G cannula after collecting a blood sample for grouping and typing. One should not wait for the transfusion. Resuscitation of the patient and surgery should be performed immediately. Laparotomy is performed under general anesthesia. As soon as the peritoneal cavity is opened the uterus is lifted up and tubes and ovaries are examined. The affected tube is picked up and clamped at either end (isthmic and infundibulo-pelvic ligament) to arrest bleeding from the tube. If blood is not readily available, autotransfusion of peritoneal blood can be arranged by collecting the peritoneal blood and filtering it into a sterile bottle containing citrate solution and transfusing it back into the patient. Salpingectomy is performed in most of the cases. Blood is sucked out or mopped and the peritoneal cavity is washed with saline. If the tube is not badly damaged and she is a nullipara, a salpingostomy could be done. Intraoperative transfusions may be used as needed. Postoperatively oral antibiotics (ampicillin 500 mg orally qid for 3–4 days) and hematinics for 3–4 months are indicated.

Follow up

When laparoscopic salpingostomy is done, and in cases of medical management, the patient has to be followed up until the β-hCG level returns to non-pregnant levels (e.g. < 3 iu/l). In case she is Rh-negative, anti-D immunisation is needed.

Though chances of subsequent intrauterine pregnancy going on to term are about 66 per cent, there is also an 8–10 per cent risk of recurrent ectopic pregnancy in these women. Therefore, as soon as she misses her period the next time, intrauterine gestation has to be confirmed by USG and tubal pregnancy has to be ruled out.

Bibliography

Anne N et al 2001. Follow-up after surgical treatment for tubal pregnancy. *Fertil Steril* 75: 560–68.

Bagshawe KD 1976. Risk and prognostic factors in trophoblastic neoplasia. *Cancer* 38: 1373–85.

Bongso TA and **Lim J** 2003. Genetics and Infertility. In SS Ratnam, KB Rao, S Arulkumaran (eds) *Obstetrics and Gynecology for Postgraduates*, vol 2, second edn. Chennai: Orient Longman.

Carr DH 1971. Chromosome and abortion. In H Harris and K Hirschorn (eds) *Advances in Human Genetics*. New York: Plenum Press, 201–51.

Curry SL and **Hammond CB** 1975. H. mole: Diagnosis, management and long term follow up. *Obstet Gynecol* 45: 1–8.

Flystra D 1998. Review of current diagnosis and treatment of tubal pregnancy. *Obstet Gynecol Surv* 53: 320–28.

Gindier J, **Li Z** and **Berry R** 2001. Folic acid supplements in pregnancy and risk of miscarriage. *Lancet* 358: 796–800.

Goldberg AB, **Greenberg MB** and **Darney PD** 2001. Misoprostol in pregnancy. *N Engl J Med* 344: 38–47.

Lipscomb GH, **Stovall TG**, and **Ling FW** 2000. Non-surgical treatment of ectopic gestation. *N Engl J Med* 343: 325–29.

Mukherjee SN 1999. The abortion problem. In SS Ratnam, KB Rao, S Arulkumaran (eds) *Obstetrics and Gynecology for Postgraduates*, vol 1, second edn. Chennai: Orient Longman, 214–27.

Newlands ES and **Bagshawe KD** 1986. Chemotherapy for medium and high risk gestational tumors. *Br J Obstet Gynecol* 3: 63–69.

Rao KB 1999. Trophoblastic tumours. In KB Rao and NN Roy Choudhury (eds) *Clinical Gynecology*, fourth edn. Chennai: Orient Longman, 180–86.

Sowter MC, **Farquhar CM** et al 2001. A randomised trial comparing single dose systemic methotrexate and laparoscopic surgery for the treatment of unruptured tubal pregnancy. *Br J Obstet Gynecol* 108: 192–203.

Tham KF and Ratnam SS 1999. Trophoblastic disease in reproductive tract. In SS Ratnam, KB Rao, S Arulkumaran (eds) *Obstetrics and Gynecology for Postgraduates*, vol 1, second edn. Chennai: Orient Longman, 352–63.

Yang J and Savitz DA 2001. Effect of vaginal bleeding in pregnancy on preterm births. *Pediatr Perinat Epidemiol* 15: 34–36.

3. Emergency contraception

Emergency contraception is the use of contraception after unprotected sexual intercourse (using contraception as a hindsight method). It is also called postcoital contraception or the morning-after pill.

Its use has led to the prevention of thousands of unwanted pregnancies and unsafe abortions thus contributing to reduction of maternal mortality and morbidity. This method is also extremely useful in cases of rape.

Methods of emergency contraception

The following methods may be used:

1. ***Levonorgestrel:*** Levonorgestrel 750 mg given orally in two doses at intervals of 12 hours or as a single dose of 1.5 mg, gives over 90 per cent protection. The earlier it is taken after the event, the better the effect. Though effective when used within 72 hours, the best results are obtained when used within 12 hours.
2. ***Yuzpe's method:*** Two oral contraceptive pills (each with estrogen content of 50 μg ethinyl estradiol) are given, at a time, in intervals of 12 hours (total 4 tablets). It is more effective when taken early and has to be taken with 3 days of exposure. The incidence of nausea and vomiting is high with this method.
3. ***Mifepristone (RU 486):*** This is an antiprogestin. Earlier 600 mg was advised orally and it was found to be as

effective as levonorgestrel. A recent WHO trial has showed that even a smaller dose of 10 mg of RU 486 is effective in preventing pregnancy in 98.5 per cent of cases.

4. ***Intrauterine copper releasing device:*** This too serves as emergency contraception if inserted within 5 days of unprotected intercourse. However, it cannot be used in a nullipara because of the difficulty of insertion in addition to the risk of infection.

If postcoital contraception should fail and pregnancy is detected later, the unwanted pregnancy could be terminated.

Pregnancy less than 49 days duration

1. Administer 600 mg of mifepristone orally followed 48 hours later by oral misoprostol 800 mg. This has 95 per cent success rate.
2. Alternatively, she could be given methotrexate 50 mg IM followed 48 hours later by oral misoprostol 800 mg.

A week later if the pregnancy has not aborted and the pregnancy test is positive, vacuum curettage is done.

In case of rape victims, smears and serological tests for STD are taken for appropriate treatment if any of the tests prove positive.

Contraception is an important component of reproductive health. It is necessary to prevent pregnancies too early (< 18 years), too late (> 35 years), too close (< 2 years) and too many, and also to prevent unwanted pregnancies.

Methods of contraception

Different methods of contraception are available (Table 3.1) (Kubba 2000). The choice of contraceptive depends upon age, parity, lactation, associated diseases (such as hypertension, cardiovascular disease, DUB, myoma), previous history of thromboembolism, breast cancer, smoking history, and whether contraception is for occasional or regular use.

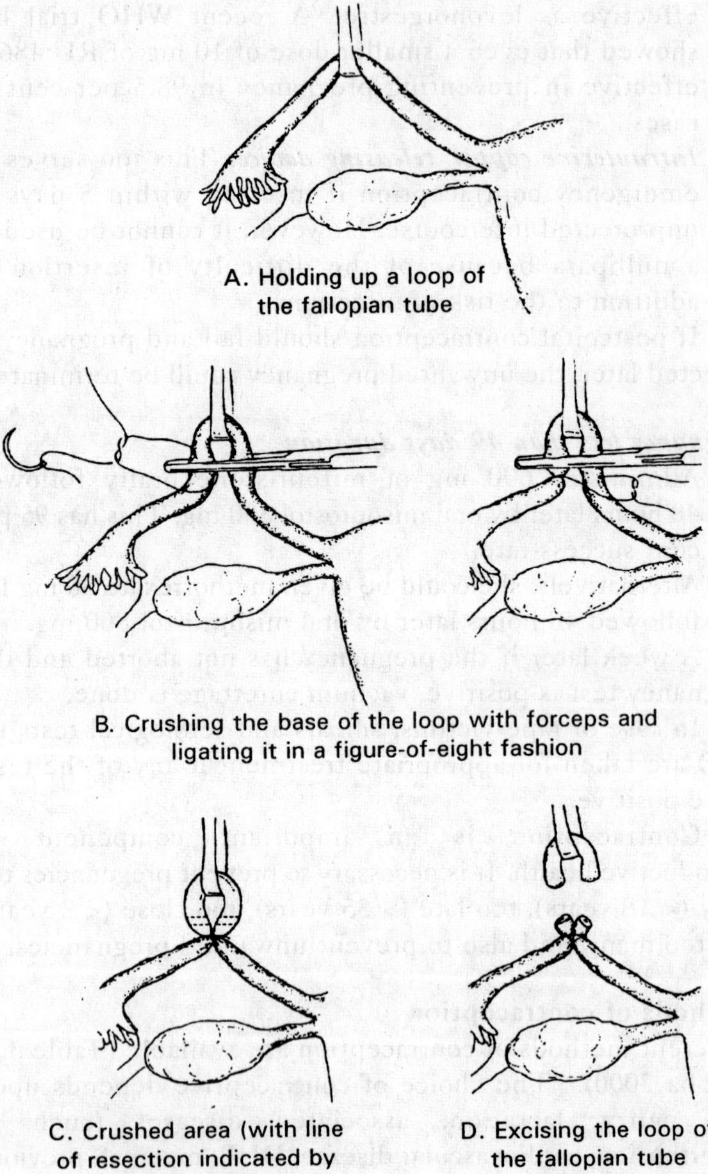

Fig 3.1 Tubal ligation

Table 3.1: Different methods of contraception currently in use

Method	*Advantages*	*Disadvantages / Contraindications*	*Failure rate at the end of 1 yr (per cent)*
Hormonal OCP, Combined	Nullipara, DUB	Thromboembolism, smoker, cancer breast	0.1
Depot DMPA	Breast-feeding Multipara	BTB, weight gain	0.3
Subdermal implant	Long term use	As above	0.05
IUCD CuT/380-a	Multipara Long term use Breast-feeding Concurrently with MTP	Infection, myoma, menorrhagia, previous ectopic	0.6
LNG 20	Perimenopausal use, DUB		0.1
Condom, male	Protects against HIV/PID	Allergy	5
Cervical cap	Waiting for other methods		9 (nullipara) 26 (multipara)
Symptothermal	Other methods cannot be used		2
Vasectomy	Permanent		0.5
Tubectomy*	methods		0.1

Source: Adapted from Kubba, 2000
* Fig 3.1

BIBLIOGRAPHY

ACOG 2001. Emergency contraception. *ACOG Prac Bull* 25.

Kubba A 2000. Contraception. *Lancet* 356: 1913–19.

Von Hertren H, Piaggio G et al 2002. Mifepristone and levonergestrel for emergency contraception: A WHO trial. *Lancet* 360: 1803–10.

WHO 1998. WHO task force on postovulatory methods of fertility control. *Lancet* 343: 428–33.

4. Hypertensive disorders of pregnancy

PREGNANCY INDUCED HYPERTENSION

Pregnancy induced hypertension (PIH) is hypertension noticed after 20 weeks of pregnancy, during labour and/or within 48 hours after delivery. Hypertension means a diastolic blood pressure (DBP) of 90 mmHg or more when recorded on two occasions four hours apart.

Preeclampsia is a multisystem disorder characterised by hypertension and proteinuria. It may be mild or severe. In the severe type the DBP is above 110 mmHg and protein levels in urine exceed 5 g in 24 h. Preeclampsia with convulsions is called eclampsia. PIH may progress to severe preeclampsia and eclampsia. It is responsible for 13 per cent of all maternal deaths in developing countries.

Incidence

It is about 8 per cent, but the severe forms, as eclampsia may be seen in 1 in 100 to 1 in 1500 deliveries depending on the quality of prenatal care.

Etiology

This is not clearly understood. The placental factor responsible for vasospasm (hypertension) and the cause of endothelial injury in multiple organs like liver, kidneys, brain, vascular system is not known.

The predisposing factors associated with PIH include nulliparity, diabetes, multiple pregnancy, chronic hypertension, renal disease, extremes of reproductive age (below 16 years or above 35 years), maternal obesity, thrombophilia and previous history of PIH.

Signs, symptoms and diagnosis

In PIH, the only sign is hypertension. Proteinuria may be present, but it may also be seen in pyelitis or fevers. Edema is not considered a useful finding as it may be noticed in over a third of normal pregnant women in the last trimester, and also in those with anemia or heart disease complicating pregnancy. In severe preeclampsia, besides DBP of over 110 mmHg and significant proteinuria, the patient may complain of headache, blurred vision, epigastric pain and oliguria (less than 400 ml in 24 h) and show evidence of pulmonary edema and marked thrombocytopenia (< 100,000/ml). This condition is called imminent eclampsia.

Sometimes the first presentation of severe preeclampsia may be with convulsions without any preceding warning symptoms. Therefore a case of severe preeclampsia must be treated on the same lines as eclampsia.

Differential diagnosis: Differential diagnosis could be (Table 4.1):

1. Essential hypertension
2. Epilepsy
3. Tetanus
4. Cerebral malaria
5. Meningitis

Prognosis and complications

Maternal complications

1. HELLP syndrome: hemolysis, elevated liver enzymes, low platelet counts with a risk of maternal death in 20 per cent.
2. Cerebral hemorrhage is the commonest post mortem finding in severe PIH.

Table 4.1: Differential diagnosis of eclampsia

Condition	*Typical signs and symptoms*	*Similarity to PIH*
Essential hypertension	BP > 130/90 before 20 weeks Superimposed preeclampsia	Mid-pregnancy drop followed by superimposed PIH
Epilepsy	BP normal History of aura and fits before pregnancy	Convulsions with coma
Tetanus	Trismus Abdominal rigidity Opsitotonus Conscious during fits	Convulsions
Cerebral malaria	Fever with rigor Anemia Spleen palpable Blood smear is diagnostic	Convulsions with coma
Meningitis	Neck rigidity Photophobia Fever	Convulsions with coma

3. Acute renal failure due to cortical necrosis
4. Pulmonary complications like pneumonia and edema

Maternal mortality in severe PIH is about 5 per cent.

Fetal complications

1. IUGR
2. Low birth weight
3. Intrauterine death

The perinatal mortality in severe PIH is about 15 per cent.

Treatment

Preventive: Currently no preventive therapy is available against PIH even though aspirin, calcium, magnesium and fish oil have been tried.

Management of PIH is mainly aimed at

1. Good control of blood pressure
2. Prevention and control of convulsions
3. Delivering the mother near term

Once the uterus is emptied, she recovers as the BP returns to normal.

Mild PIH

Rest and oral sedation if required. No hypotensives are required. The BP is recorded twice daily as an outpatient. If the BP returns to normal she is managed as a normal pregnancy. If, however, the condition remains as mild PIH with no proteinuria, labour is induced close to the expected date of delivery (EDD) depending on the nature of the cervix. If the cervix is ripe, amniotomy and oxytocin drip is preferred. If not, endocervical PGE_2 should be used, followed if necessary with amniotomy; oxytocin infusion may also be tried.

The higher the DBP, the greater the risk of eclampsia. Therefore, in all cases of PIH, the blood pressure has to be monitored during labour. The second stage of labour is cut short with a forceps if necessary. Ergometrine has to be avoided during the third stage of labour as it may raise the BP further. If needed, oxytocin 20 units could be used in 500 ml of 5% dextrose IV to prevent PPH.

Severe preeclampsia: The patient should be hospitalised and treated actively as in eclampsia. The obstetric management of severe PIH prior to 33 weeks is a challenge to the physician who has to choose between the risks to the mother and her fetus.

Conservative management may benefit the fetus but will increase maternal morbidity. In institutions with good intensive neonatal care facilities, the management decision may be easier.

1. Control of BP: In severe cases of PIH the DBP should be brought down to 90 mmHg to prevent convulsions and cerebral hemorrhage. The hypotensive of choice is hydrallazine, given in a dose of 10–15 mg IV slowly. If BP is still high it could be repeated in 10 mg doses every 15–30 minutes. The daily dose should not exceed 100 mg.

The calcium antagonist nifedipine could be tried in 5–10 mg doses sublingually. It could be repeated every 15–30 minutes depending on the level of DBP. Alternatively, labetalol is used at the dose of 50 mg slow IV. If needed 60 mg can be given as an IV drip in 500 ml of Ringer lactate solution to regulate the BP. No diuretics are indicated as there is already hemoconcentration.

2. Prevention and control of convulsions: The drug of choice is magnesium sulphate ($MgSO_4$) given parenterally (Table 4.2). The MAGPIE trial (2002) has shown that parenteral magnesium sulphate given over 24 hours is the drug of choice in severe PIH for the prevention of eclampsia and significant reduction in maternal mortality.

   If it is not available, diazepam is used (10 mg IV as a bolus slowly). If required an additional 10 mg is given, followed by 40 mg in 500 ml of Ringer lactate solution as IV drip to keep the patient well-sedated but arousable to mild painful stimulus. The total dose must not exceed 100 mg in 24 hours. Diazepam produces respiratory depression in the mother and causes hypotonia and respiratory depression in the fetus and therefore should be the second choice after $MgSO_4$.

Table 4.2: Magnesium sulphate therapy for severe PIH including eclampsia

Loading dose: 4 g of 20% magnesium sulphate solution is given slowly (over 5 min). This is immediately followed with 5 g of 50% solution IM in each buttock deep into the muscle. If convulsions recur within 15 minutes repeat 2 g IV of 20% solution.
Maintenance dose: 5 g of 50% solution 4 hourly into alternate buttock for 24 h after delivery.
Caution: If respiratory rate is less than 12 per min, patellar reflexes are absent or if the hourly urinary output is less than 30 ml, withold the injection. Antidote is 10 ml of 10% calcium gluconate IV

3. Obstetric management: If the patient responds to treatment, the delivery is conducted 24 hours later depending on the period of gestation and the cervical condition. If the cervix is ripe, amniotomy and oxytocin should be the choice.

CASE REPORT 1

An unbooked 24-year-old primigravida, 8 months pregnant was admitted as an emergency with history of headache followed by two fits an hour earlier. On examination she was drowsy, restless and had edema on both legs. Her BP was 160/96 mmHg. She was started on eclampsia therapy with $MgSO_4$ parenterally (Table 4.2). Abdominal examination showed the uterus to be 30 weeks in size; there were no contractions; the head was floating and the FH sounds were normal. On catheterisation 200 ml of urine (albumin ++) was drained. She responded to treatment as there were no more convulsions. However, as the BP was still fluctuating between 140/90 and 160/100 mmHg and the risk of recurrence of fits was still present, a cesarean section was advised. She was given betamethazone 12 mg IM twice at 12 hour intervals prior to the cesarean section. The baby weighed 1.6 kg and was looked after by the neonatologist. The BP was within normal limits from the third postoperative day.

This case of antepartum eclampsia could have been prevented if the patient had had proper prenatal care. The earlier the onset of PIH or preeclampsia, the worse the prognosis. Though she responded to anticonvulsant therapy, she was only 30 weeks, not in labour with high BP and a possibility of recurrence of fits. Cesarean section was the appropriate management.

Cesarean section is indicated in severe PIH/eclampsia:

- If the cervix is not ripe
- An eclamptic is restless and not responding to therapy

- If labour is likely to be delayed
- In severe IUGR
- In cases of fetal distress
- If there is any evidence of vaginal bleeding with or without tenderness of the uterus (abruptio placentae) with a live fetus.

In a large muticentre study of over 1200 eclampsia cases, the cesarean section rate was over 66 per cent (Eclampsia Trial Group 1995). Anticonvulsant therapy is continued for 48 hours after the delivery. The BP is monitored till it remains normal. If it is high even after the puerperium she is classified as a case of essential hypertension and treated accordingly.

If necessary the patient is referred to the tertiary hospital in cases of HELLP syndrome, severe oliguria or anuria, coagulation failure, coma for more than 12 hours, localising neurological signs or status eclampticus.

ESSENTIAL HYPERTENSION IN PREGNANCY

When pregnancy occurs in a known hypertensive or when hypertension is noticed in a pregnant woman prior to 20 weeks, it is known as essential hypertension.

Incidence

About 10–15 per cent of all pregnancies; mostly in multiparous women or in the diabetic pregnant women.

Signs and symptoms

In all these women BP is raised. Some of them may have symptoms due to cardiac decompensation as a result of chronic hypertension or secondary renal pathology. As pregnancy advances the BP may rise but most of them show a mid-pregnancy drop to normal levels, and later (after 20 weeks) display hypertension alone (which may be mistaken for PIH) or with superimposed preeclampsia.

In a person with mild hypertension, the BP may be less than 160/110. However, in severe hypertension it may be over

160–180/110–120 mmHg. It is advisable that in chronic hypertension examination and laboratory investigations be done to find out the status of the heart, kidneys as well as the eye at the beginning of pregnancy or even prior to it. This helps in monitoring effects of the pregnancy on these organs.

Diagnosis

Elevated BP before 20 weeks merely establishes the diagnosis of a hypertensive disorder in pregnancy. It is necessary to find out whether it is only essential hypertension or it is of renal, adrenal, autoimmune (e.g. SLE), vascular or due to thyroid disease. One has also to find out to what extent the heart and other organs are affected as a result of it.

Complications and prognosis

Maternal complications

1. Cerebral hemorrhage
2. Superimposed preeclampsia and eclampsia
3. Abruptio placentae
4. Cardiac failure
5. Renal failure

Fetal complications

These include IUGR, prematurity and intrauterine death.

Treatment

Mild cases only need monitoring of BP and fetal growth. The patient could be allowed to deliver at term. There is no need for hypotensives. If she was taking hypotensive drugs prior to pregnancy it could be continued if it is not teratogenic or contraindicated in pregnancy.

The Appendix describes the management of a hypertensive emergency.

Severe cases of chronic hypertension

Such patients always require antihypertensives to prevent complications. The BP should be maintained within reasonably safe levels (and not brought down to normal) to allow perfusion of the kidneys and the placenta. The most commonly used hypotensives are methyldopa 500 mg qid, or labetalol an alpha- and beta-blocker. Atenolol and other beta-blockers may cause the newborn to be small for gestational age (SGA). Calcium antagonists like nifedipine could be used. ACE inhibitors are considered teratogenic and could cause renal, facial and other defects.

If preeclampsia is noticed, it is treated depending on whether it is mild or severe, as stated earlier under PIH. The pregnancy is terminated in the presence of the following indications:

1. Severe preeclampsia any time after 28 weeks depending on its effect on the mother/fetus
2. Mild preeclampsia by 37 weeks
3. Severe IUGR
4. Abruptio placentae
5. HELLP syndrome

In these cases depending on the maternal and fetal condition, period of gestation and the favourability of the cervix, amniotomy and oxytocin infusion or prostaglandin induction or cesarean section may have to be chosen to terminate the pregnancy.

After the delivery they should be followed up to provide advice regarding future childbearing and the need for surveillance of the hypertension.

Bibliography

ACOG 2001. Chronic hypertension in pregnancy. *Prac Bull* 29.

Eclampsia Trial Group 1995. Which is the best anticonvulsant for eclampsia? *Lancet* 345: 1455–63.

Garovic VD 2000. Hypertension in pregnancy. *Mayo Clin Proc* 75: 1071–76.

The MAGPIE Trial Collaborative Group 2002. Do women with preeclampsia benefit from magnesium sulphate? *Lancet* 359: 1877–90.

Walker JJ 2001. Severe PIH and eclampsia. *Bailliere's Clin Obstet Gynecol* vol 4, 59–71.

5. Hemorrhages in late pregnancy and labour

Hemorrhage in late pregnancy is described as hemorrhage from the genital tract after 20 weeks of gestation and before the birth of the baby.

Incidence
About 2 per cent of all deliveries.

Etiology
There are two important causes:

1. Hemorrhage due to premature separation of a normally implanted placenta (in the upper uterine segment). It is called abruptio placentae or accidental hemorrhage. It is usually due to PIH. However, it may follow trauma (fall or blunt injury over the abdomen), or sudden decompression of the uterus (as with rupture of membranes in polyhydramnios). The bleeding in this condition may be revealed, concealed or mixed.
2. Hemorrhage due to separation of an abnormally implanted placenta (in the lower uterine segment); it is also called placenta previa (Fig 5.1). In such cases the placenta is partly or fully covering the cervical os. Bleeding is inevitable (and recurrent) as the placenta is separated when there is elongation of the lower uterine segment as pregnancy advances or as the cervix dilates in labour. It is always revealed or external.

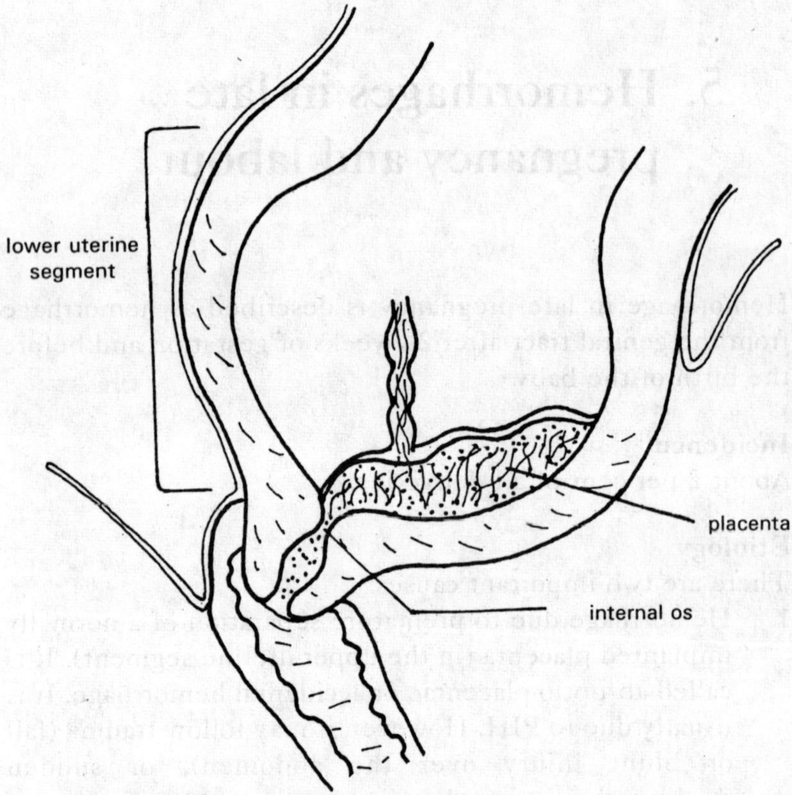

Fig 5.1 Placenta in the lower segment

The bleeding may, in rare cases, be due to cervical polyp or cancer or due to vasa previa. Occasionally, the bleeding in labour may be due to rupture of the uterus (chapter 7). Abruptio placentae is more common in India as compared to other south Asian countries.

ABRUPTIO PLACENTAE

Diagnosis

In abruptio placentae, the patient is often a primipara with PIH. For diagnostic and prognostic purposes the condition is classified into four grades.

Grade 0 The patient is asymptomatic, but after the delivery a retroplacental clot is seen.

Grade 1 There is slight, vaginal bleeding; her general condition is normal and there is no evidence of fetal distress. USG shows placenta in its normal site with evidence of slight separation at its lower margin.

Grade 2 External bleeding may or may not be seen; uterine tenderness with tetany and fetal distress are present (mixed type).

Grade 3 There may be slight or no external bleeding and yet she may look pale with evidence of shock. The uterus is tense, woody (hard) and tender, with no fetal heart on auscultation. These cases do not warrant a USG but if performed, may reveal gross disruption of chorio-decidual space with retro-placental clots and no FH activity. In about a third of these patients coagulopathy is noticed.

Differential diagnosis

Differential diagnosis is rupture of the uterus or anemia with acute polyhydramnios (Table 5.1).

In no case of antepartum hemorrhage should a digital vaginal examination be performed except in an institution with the blood bank and operation theatre ready.

Complications and prognosis

Complications are i) shock, ii) uterine inertia, iii) PPH, iv) DIC with coagulation failure, and v) acute renal failure. Maternal mortality is 2–3 per cent. Perinatal mortality is about 40 per cent.

Table 5.1: Differential diagnosis of abruptio placentae

Diagnosis	*Typical Findings*
Abruptio placentae, concealed tube	Pale, shock +, uterus tender and woody, FH absent, no vaginal bleeding
Rupture uterus	Pale, shock +, uterine outline absent, fetal parts easily felt, no FH, vaginal bleeding +
Anemia with polyhydramnios	Pale, no shock, uterus overdistended, tense, fluid thrill +, FH ±, no vaginal bleeding
Placenta previa	Pale, shock ±, uterus lax, malpresentation or head floating high, FH +, vaginal bleeding ±

Management

1. On admission, check hemoglobin, blood group and Rh type (if not checked earlier).
2. Treat shock, if present (chapter 18); start normal saline or Ringer lactate IV.
3. Alert the blood bank.
4. Check clotting time (normal 7 minutes) and clot retraction time (a stable clot is formed in 20 minutes).
5. Ascertain the amount of blood loss (from pads/external bleeding, uterine tenderness and distension, if any) and replace blood loss.
6. Find out period of gestation, fetal size (weight) and condition. If the fetus is viable and shows evidence of distress, immediate delivery should be undertaken. Determine the placental site with ultrasonography, as described earlier (pp 37).

If pregnancy is less than 36 weeks, there is no PIH or bleeding and the general condition is good, perform a speculum examination to rule out cervical causes of bleeding. Wait till 36 weeks and intervene only if a moderate bout of bleeding occurs.

If the pregnancy is over 36 weeks and if there is bleeding, she is examined in the theatre—if the cervix admits a finger and membranes are felt, then amniotomy and oxytocin drip is started. She is monitored for any bleeding (including clotting and clot reaction time at intervals), pulse/ BP and CTG. If the labour progresses satisfactorily, after the baby is born, check the amount of retroplacental clots.

Note that in all cases of APH, whether the delivery is vaginal or by cesarean section, PPH must be minimised by using IV ergometrine (which is withheld if her BP is raised) and oxytocin 20 units in IV drip. If atonic PPH persists carboprost (15 methyl PGF_{2a}) 250 µg is given IM and repeated 15 minutes later, if needed (case report 1, chapter 15).

Cesarean section in abruptio placentae is indicated in:
1. Fetal distress (persistent bradycardia /deceleration)
2. Signs of hemodynamic disturbance
3. Persistent bleeding in spite of amniotomy and oxytocin infusion
4. Uterine inertia with delivery unlikely in the next 2–3 hours
5. Multipara with bad obstetric history

Cesarean section is reported in about 40 per cent of cases.

Treatment of complications

1. In severe types of concealed abruptio placentae, after the cesarean section the uterus may show blotches of subserosal bleeding as the hemorrhage appears to have ploughed through the myometrium. In a few of these cases of Couvelaire uterus where atonic PPH may persist in spite of oxytocics as advised earlier, a subtotal hysterectomy may be life saving.
2. Coagulation failure: If coagulation failure is detected, it should be corrected promptly with adequate fresh whole blood transfusion. If not available, the clotting factors should be replaced by the following:
   - Fresh frozen plasma 15 ml/kg (1 litre or 4 units)
   - Packed RBCs
   - Cryoprecipitate 10 units. If platelet count is low (< 50 000/ml) platelet concentrate is advised.

   If in a case of acute renal failure, anuria persists for

24 hours even after the shock is treated, she should be transferred to a tertiary level centre for further management.

PLACENTA PREVIA

In placenta previa the patient is usually a multipara, in the last trimester, complaining of painless, recurrent and causeless bleeding. Her general condition (and of her child) depends on the amount of external blood loss. The uterus is lax with the fetal head floating high up or there is a malpresentation like breech presentation (Fig 5.2). USG is extremely useful not only in the diagnosis of this condition but also to find out if the placenta is fully or partly covering the os.

Management

This depends on her general condition, presence of active bleeding and on the condition and maturity of the fetus. If the gestation is less than 36 weeks, there is no or minimal bleeding and no labour pains, adopt a conservative

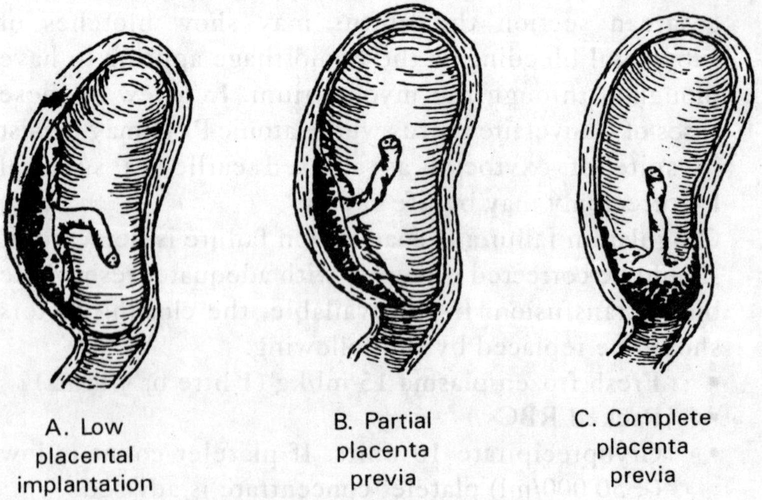

Fig 5.2 Placenta previa

management to improve chances of fetal survival. The patient's hemoglobin and blood type is checked (as described under abruptio placentae).

Active management with immediate intervention is needed if

- there is moderate to severe bleeding
- she goes into premature labour and
- the fetus is mature.

The best results are obtained for both the mother and her child by doing cesarean section in all cases of placenta previa (given an indication for delivery). The exception to this is when the placenta is anterior and is of the marginal type. In such a case, in the theatre, an amniotomy and oxytocin infusion is tried. Even here, if bleeding persists cesarean section is indicated. Since the vascular lower segment cannot contract and retract (like the upper segment) in the third stage, steps must always be taken to minimise PPH as stated earlier. If during a cesarean section the anterior lower segment is found to be very vascular these vessels could be sutured before cutting the lower segment. In a multipara, under such a rare condition, classical cesarean and tubal sterilisation is safer. Occasionally, in a case of previous cesarean, the placenta may be morbidly adherent (as placenta accreta), when hysterectomy may be necessary.

If a patient with antepartum hemorrhage is admitted in a state of shock, resuscitate her first and if she is not in labour, deliver her using cesarean section. It is extremely important that in such cases PPH be prevented.

BIBLIOGRAPHY

Biswas A and Arulkumaran S 1999. Antepartum hemorrhage. In SS Ratnam, KB Rao and S Arulkumaran S (Eds) *Obstetrics and Gynecology for Postgraduates*, 2nd edn, Madras: Orient Longman, 78–88.

Droste S and Kiel K 1994. Expectant management of placenta previa. *Am J Obstet Gynecol* 170: 1254–57.

Lavery J P 1990 Placenta previa. *Clin Obstet Gynecol* 33: 414–20.

6. Emergencies in late pregnancy: preterm labour, PROM and absence of fetal movements

PRETERM LABOUR

Preterm labour is defined as onset of labour after 22 weeks of gestation but before 37 weeks of pregnancy. Preterm delivery accounts for over 50 per cent of all neonatal deaths and significant neonatal morbidity. In addition, 10 per cent of those born before 28 weeks of pregnancy will be severely handicapped.

Incidence

Incidence is 8–10 per cent of all pregnancies.

Causes

1. Anemias and toxemias of pregnancy
2. Overdistension of the uterus, twins, hydramnios
3. Bacterial vaginosis
4. Malpresentations like breech
5. Fetal anomalies
6. Internal os insufficiency

Risk factors for preterm labour include:

1. Demographic factors like age less than 17 years and over

35 years; low socioeconomic status, low pre-pregnancy weight
2. History of preterm birth, especially in the second trimester, and history of vaginal bleeding in more than one trimester
3. Smoking

Diagnosis

This can be diagnosed from the history and from clinical findings. Abdominal palpation confirms preterm size of the uterus and painful intermittent uterine contractions. One may also guess at the probable cause (such as malpresentations or multiple pregnancies). The fetal heart is also checked. In some women 'show' or bloodstained mucoid vaginal discharge may be present. Ultrasonography may help confirm the premature gestation and find out the possible cause of preterm labour, such as polyhydramnios or multiple pregnancy.

Biological markers

Biological markers for predicting preterm birth are:
1. Salivary estriol estimations: Adrenal production of dihydroepiandrosterone (DHEA) increases the placental synthesis of estrogen as a result of which levels of maternal serum estradiol and salivary estriol increase before the onset of spontaneous or premature labour. However, as the test carries a high false positive rate it is not very reliable.
2. Bacterial vaginosis is associated with premature labour, but large trials have failed to show the correlation (Morris 2001).
3. Fetal fibronectin (fFN) is produced by fetal membranes. It helps to bind the placenta and membranes to the decidua. The presence of fFN in cervical secretions after 20 weeks of gestation is an indicator of impending preterm labour especially when it is associated with the

cervical length of 2.5 cm or less when measured by ultrasonography.

Management

The patient is advised rest and treatment. The aim of the treatment should be:

1. To arrest or delay labour and to gain time for corticosteroids to act. Each day's delay would mean reduction of chances of neonatal mortality.
2. To treat the cause, if any.

Tocolytics are used to arrest labour when

- Gestation is less than 34 weeks
- Cervix is dilated to less than 3 cm
- There is no amnionitis
- There is no fetal distress

If the gestation is less than 37 weeks, betamethasone 12 mg IM is given twice at an interval of 12 hours to help lung maturation in the fetus. This need not be repeated even if the child is not born within a week of the injection. However, glucocorticoids are not beneficial if the gestation is less than 28 weeks.

The drugs used are:

1. Salbutamol 5 mg in 500 ml of 5% dextrose at 10 drops/min raised every half hour by 10 drops till contractions stop. Later, maintain the rate for 48 hours. Stop infusion in case of any maternal tachycardia (pulse rate above 120/min), palpitation, chest discomfort or pain, dyspnea (pulmonary edema) or fetal distress.
2. Magnesium sulphate IM
3. Nifedipine 5–10 mg orally
4. An oxytocin antagonist, atosiban. Atosiban is given IV as an initial bolus dose of 6.75 mg. Later give 300 μg/min IV for 3 hours and maintain at 100 μg/min thereafter for 48 hours. Recent trials have shown that atosiban is as effective as a beta-mimetic drug, and has fewer side effects. To inhibit preterm labour, atosiban or nifedipine

are the drugs of choice as they have the least adverse effects.

If speculum examination and study of the vaginal smear show bacterial vaginosis, metronidazole 400 mg bid for a week or a single dose of 2 g is given. Metronidazole 0.75% gel could also be used vaginally. Though the use of metronidazole is claimed to be useful in cases of preterm labour, randomised clinical trials have shown that it is useful only in patients with a previous history of preterm labour. The Oracle 1 study has shown that prophylactic antibiotics are useful in preterm labour.

The pregnancy may be allowed to progress if
- Cervical dilatation is 4 cm or more
- Period of gestation is close to 37 weeks
- Presence of APH, PIH or any fetal distress is noted

Vacuum extraction is avoided in case of preterm delivery. (See chapter 14 for care of the premature baby)

PRELABOUR RUPTURE OF MEMBRANES (PROM)

Prelabour rupture of membranes (PROM) indicates rupture of the bag of membranes prior to the onset of labour. PROM may take place at term (after 37 weeks of pregnancy). When it occurs before 37 weeks, that is, prematurely between 22 and 37 weeks, it is called premature PROM (PPROM). PPROM is an important cause of premature delivery and increased perinatal morbidity and mortality. It also contributes to amnionitis and maternal morbidity.

Incidence
About 1–1.5 per cent of deliveries.

Etiology
Among the causes discussed under preterm labour, infections, especially bacterial vaginosis with organisms like mycoplasma,

ureaplasma, and gardnerella are important causes. Other organisms may also cause amnionitis and lead to rupture of the membranes at the point of weakness. The prostaglandins released endocervically may also initiate preterm labour.

Diagnosis

PROM is suspected from the woman's history of vaginal watery discharge, and by noting that the pad given to her is wet. Speculum examination will show watery discharge from the cervix particularly when she is asked to cough. It could be confirmed as liquor amni by the nitrazine test or the fern test.

Nitrazine test: When the nitrazine paper dipped into a drop of liquor turns from yellow to blue it proves the alkalinity of this fluid

Fern test: When a drop of this fluid is taken on a glass slide, allowed to dry and examined under the microscope, a fern pattern is seen.

In these cases ultrasonography may be helpful; check if there has been any reduction in the volume of liquor. Besides, it can also indicate the maturity of the fetus and detect fetal anomaly.

In cases of PROM repeat vaginal examination is not performed for fear of introducing infection.

Prognosis

In PPROM there is an average latency period of 1–2 weeks before the onset of labour.

Fetal prognosis

This depends on the gestation at which PROM occurred and the gestation at which delivery took place. The following figures for prognosis applies to early preterm period (less than 28 weeks). Pulmonary hypoplasia is seen in 10–30 per cent, skeletal deformities in 5 per cent, neurological or developmental defects due to prematurity and anoxia in over 60 per cent, neonatal sepsis in 10 per cent and perinatal mortality is seen in 40–50 per cent.

Maternal prognosis

Chorioamnionitis is reported in 30–40 per cent of PPROM cases.

Management

Management depends on the period of gestation and whether there is evidence of infection or amnionitis (fever, uterine tenderness and offensive vaginal discharge).

Preterm PROM: Give prophylactic antibiotics: ampicillin 500 mg tds along with erythromycin 250 mg tds orally for a week. Administer betamethasone 12 mg IM twice at an interval of 12 hours in the absence of infection. Advise bed rest and conduct delivery at or after 37 weeks.

If facilities are available, intracervical fibrin sealant is used to arrest the leakage of amniotic fluid so as to increase the liquor and help prolong the pregnancy. If there are no facilities for the care of the preterm baby in the institution, transfer the mother early to a tertiary level centre.

If the fetus is over 37 weeks' gestation, give prophylactic ampicillin 1–2 g every 6 hours if the PROM is of over 18 hours duration. If the cervix is ripe, infuse oxytocin. If the cervix is not ripe, endocervical PGE_2 followed six hours later by oxytocin infusion (if there are inadequate contractions) or misoprostol 50 mg orally every 6 hours for 3 doses could be tried. Misoprostol is not licensed for induction of labour even though when used vaginally it is more effective than conventional methods including PGE_2, and is associated with hyperstimulation of the uterus. Therefore care should be exercised to monitor the fetal condition and uterine contractions. If labour is not induced depite these measures, cesarean section should be performed.

In active management of PROM at term, oral misoprostol

50 μg, 4 hourly (with a maximum of 5 doses) may be tried or conventional methods including vaginal PGE_2 with oxytocin 24 hours later.

If the patient has amnionitis give 2 g ampicillin IV 4 times a day in addition to gentamycin 80 mg IM; depending on the nature of the cervix action is taken to deliver her.

- If the cervix is ripe infuse oxytocin.
- If it is not favourable give endocervical PGE_2 followed by oxytocin drip.

Intrauterine infection carries a major threat to the fetus and mother. Should there be any delay in delivery, cesarean section should be performed. In such cases give 500 mg metronidazole 6 hourly in addition to ampicillin, for upto two days after the patient remains afebrile.

The newborn also needs antibiotics. Culture or smear of gastric aspirate may be useful.

ABSENCE OF FETAL MOVEMENTS

A pregnant woman may complain of loss of fetal movements at any time from 22 weeks to term or during labour. It is necessary in all these cases to verify whether the fetus is alive by checking the fetal heart with a fetal stethoscope or Doppler, and to confirm it by ultrasonography. Sometimes an overanxious patient may not feel the fetal movements or the fetus may be under the effect of sedatives given to the mother. In some instances the fetus may be dead.

Incidence

The incidence of intrauterine fetal death varies from 1 to 3 per cent. The causative factors may be congenital anomalies, intrauterine infections like syphilis, PIH, diabetes, APH or, IUGR. Sometimes no cause is detectable. During labour fetal death may be due to hypoxia resulting from a hypertonic uterus, cord compression or neglected labour.

Diagnosis

Intrauterine death of the fetus could be suspected from the history of absent fetal movements or from cessation of uterine growth after the fetus dies (uterine height is less than that indicated by the period of amenorrhea). This may be confirmed by the absence of fetal heart sounds on auscultation. Ultrasonography will show absence of fetal heart and body movements, and may also show Spalding's sign (overlapping of the skull bones due to degenerative changes in the brain), doubled up fetus and absence of liquor.

Management

Gently inform the patient that the baby is dead, and explain the probable cause and its course. Reassure her and her relatives that if left alone the uterus would empty spontaneously within 3–4 weeks of fetal demise. If the mother is anxious and is keen to have the pregnancy terminated, prostaglandin induction can be offered. If after 4 weeks, it is not expelled and the platelet count and the clotting time are normal, one has to induce labour.

If vaginal examination shows a favourable cervix, oxytocin is given as a controlled drip. If it is unfavourable, vaginal PGE_2 1–2 mg or misoprostol 50 mg 6 hourly for 4 doses can be tried. In the second trimester besides vaginal misoprostol in the dose suggested earlier, instillation of 150–200 ml of ethacridine lactate solution with 250 mg of PGF_{2a} has also been found effective. In the third trimester, a dose of 100 mg of vaginal misoprostol 12 hourly has an almost 100 per cent success rate.

However, if there is evidence of coagulopathy as shown by low platelet counts and an unstable clot, the coagulation defect is corrected before emptying the uterus.

In no case should the membranes be ruptured since this may cause an infection. Cesarean section should be the last resort. Adequate pain relief and emotional support are vital.

Depending on the cause of fetal death, the mother will have to be treated to avoid its recurrence. The problem of fetal death in obstructed labour is dealt with in chapter 7.

Bibliography

ACOG 2001. Assessment of risk factors for preterm birth. *ACOG Prac Bull* 31.

Goldberg AB, Greenberg MB and Darney PD 2001. Misoprostol in pregnancy. *N Engl J Med* 344: 87–94.

Hofmeyer GJ, Gulmezoghi AM 2001. Vaginal misoprostol for cervical ripening and induction of labour in late pregnancy. Cochrane database Syst Rev 2001 (3): CD 000941.

Krishna UR and Shah M 1999. Prelabour rupture of membranes. In: Eds SS Ratnam, KB Rao and S Arulkumaran *Obstetrics and Gynecology for Postgraduates*,. Vol 1, 2nd edn. Chennai: Orient Longman, 96-107.

Lams JD, Goldenberg RL, Mercer BM et al 1998. Preterm risk study. *Am J Obstet Gynecol* 178: 1035–40.

Morris M, Nicoli N, Simms S et al 2001. Bacterial vaginosis: A review. *Br J Obstet Gynecol* 108: 439–450.

Ngai N, Chan Y, and Lam S 2000. Misoprostol vs Oxytocin in prelabour rupture of membranes. *Br J Obstet Gynecol* 107: 222–227.

Scicione AC, Manley JS, Pollok M et al 2001. Intracervical fibrin sealants for early cases of PROM. *Am J Obstet Gynecol* 184: 368–373.

Slattery MM and Morrison J 2002. Preterm delivery—review *Lancet* 360: 1489–97.

Shetty A, Stewart K et al 2002. Active management of term PROM with oral misoprostol. *Br J Obstet Gynecol* 109: 1354–58.

Wood NS, Marlow N, Costeloe K et al 2000. Neurologic and developmental disability after extremely preterm birth. *N Engl J Med* 343: 378–384.

Worldwide Atosiban Study Group 2001. Effectiveness and safety of the oxytocin antagonist atosiban versus beta adrenergic agonists in the treatment of premature labour. *Br J Obstet Gynecol* 108: 133–142.

7. Normal and abnormal labour

Normal labour may be defined as one where there is spontaneous onset of uterine contractions associated with effacement and dilatation of the cervix, and descent of the well-flexed vertex. It ends in the spontaneous birth of a healthy infant followed by expulsion of the placenta.

Incidence
In large field studies, it is about 80–82 per cent.

Diagnosis of labour
The prelabour symptoms are a feeling of lightening in the epigastric region with descent of the head into the pelvis and presence of 'show' due to dilatation of the cervix. Labour is diagnosed when there are regular painful uterine contractions with cervical changes.

The first stage of labour (from the onset of labour to full dilatation of the cervix) consists of the initial latent phase followed by an active phase. The latent phase of labour lasts for about 6–8 hours when there is cervical effacement (shortening and thinning) and dilatation to 3 cm. The active phase of labour is associated with increasing frequency and duration of uterine contractions and progressive dilatation of the cervix at the rate of 1 cm/hour from 3 cm at the beginning of active phase of labour, to full dilatation or to 10 cm (about 7 hours). The second stage of labour extends from full dilatation of cervix to the descent and complete expulsion of the baby and lasts for 1–2 hours. As the third stage does not normally exceed 10–15 minutes the total duration of normal labour is about 10–12 hours in a multipara and about 12–16 hours in a nullipara.

Management of normal labour

A woman is likely to have a normal labour if she has received antepartum education, and has a supportive attendant and a skilled professional to monitor labour.

The general principles of management are:

1. Initial assessment to determine risks, if any
2. Observing progress of labour and intervening if it is abnormal
3. Careful monitoring of fetal and maternal condition (points 2 and 3 with help of a partograph)
4. Providing pain relief, hydration and emotional support

Assessment involves eliciting a detailed history, clinical examination and asking for basic investigations such as hemoglobin, blood group and type, and testing urine for albumin and sugar. After a detailed general examination, the **abdominal examination** is performed to check

a. Frequency and duration of uterine contractions over a 10 minute period
b. Measurement of the fundal height
c. Fetal presentation and its level in relation to the pelvic brim, palpable in 'fifths' (Fig 7.1)
d. Auscultation of the fetal heart every 30 minutes in the first stage and every 5 minutes in the second stage of labour.

This is followed by **vaginal examination** to find out

a. Position, consistency, effacement and dilatation of the cervix
b. Integrity of membranes, amount and colour of liquor
c. Station of the presenting part in the pelvis (in cm) above (minus) or below (plus) the level of ischial spines (Fig 7.2)
d. Adequacy of pelvis for the childbirth

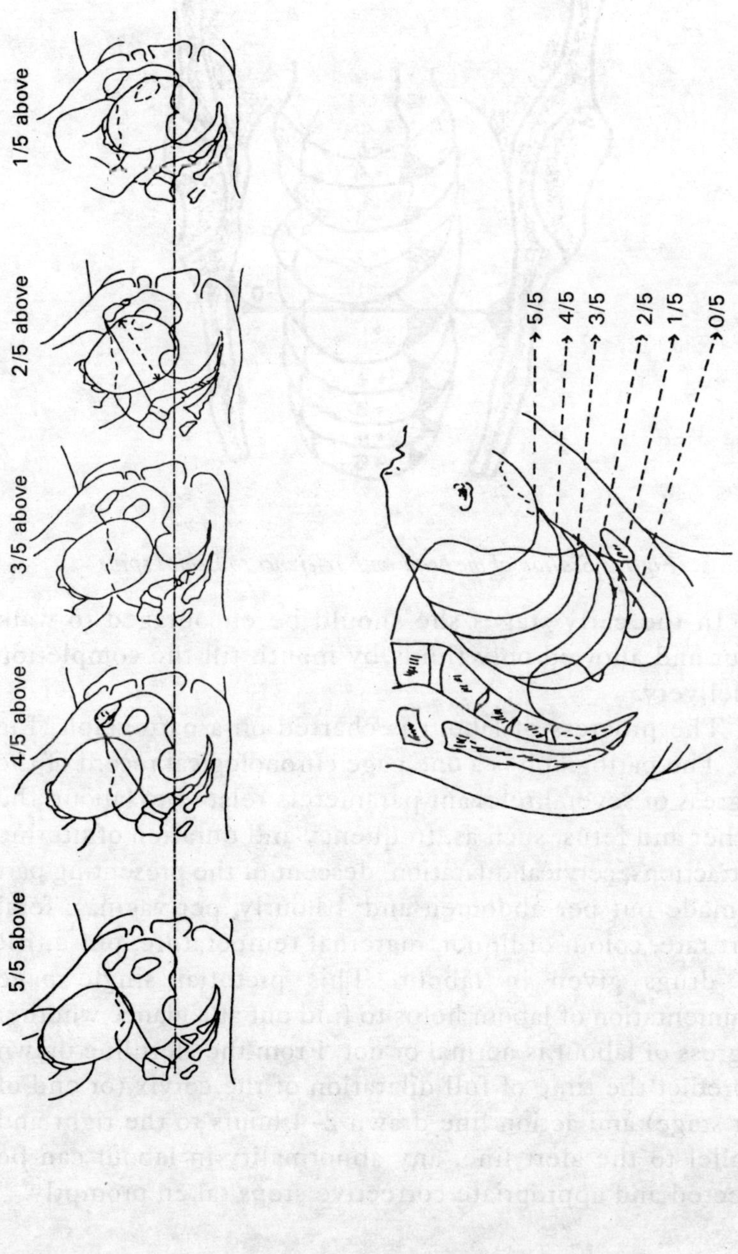

Fig 7.1 Descent of fetal head as assessed on obstetric palpation

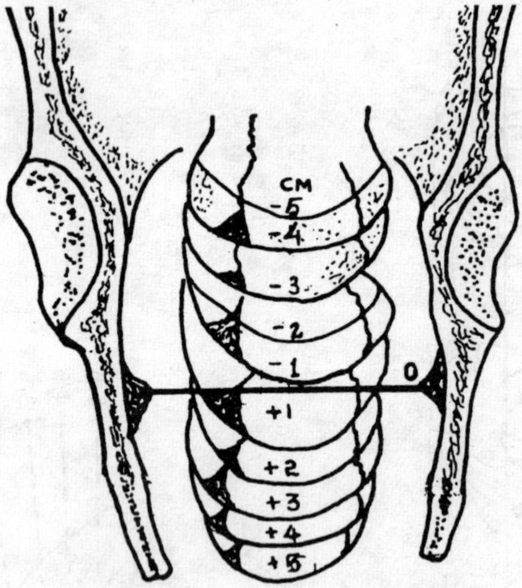

Fig 7.2 Station of the head with reference to ischial spine

In the early stages she should be encouraged to walk about and allowed only fluids by mouth till the completion of delivery.

The progress of labour is charted on a partograph (Fig 7.3). The partograph is a one page chronological record of the progress of several relevant parameters related to labour, the mother and fetus, such as, frequency and duration of uterine contractions, cervical dilatation, descent of the presenting part (as made out per abdomen and 4 hourly, per vagina), fetal heart rate, colour of liquor, maternal temperature, pulse, BP, and drugs given in labour. This pictorial single page documentation of labour helps to find out at a glance whether progress of labour is normal or not. From the alert line drawn to predict the time of full dilatation of the cervix (or end of first stage) and action line drawn 2–4 hours to the right and parallel to the alert line, any abnormality in labour can be detected and appropriate corrective steps taken promptly.

There is no particular indication or benefit in 'active management' of labour (performing an early amniotomy in the active phase routinely and following it up with oxytocin infusion to accelerate labour). Early amniotomy may be useful in selected cases like those with abnormal fetal heart rate, postdatism, PIH or IUGR to find out whether it is meconium stained.

The progress of the first stage of labour is considered poor when the rate of cervical dilatation is slower than 1 cm/hour and it extends to the right of the alert line (or expected progress line) without any appreciable descent of the presenting part. In the active first stage of labour the causes of poor progress are:

- Inefficient uterine contractions
- Fetal malposition or malpresentation
- Cephalopelvic disproportion

Management of poor progress in the first stage of labour

When the progress of labour is poor, determine its cause and treat it. The most common cause is inefficient uterine contractions; appropriate use of oxytocin to augment labour should help to achieve vaginal delivery.

Oxytocin augmentation is indicated when the cervical dilatation is less than 1 cm/hour in the active phase and the progress cuts the action line. If the membranes are still intact, amniotomy is performed. The volume and colour of the amniotic fluid should be noted. The fetal and maternal condition, as well as the uterine status are reassessed, and where facilities exist, continuous CTG recording is started. Five units of oxytocin in one litre of 5% dextrose saline or normal saline is started IV at a dose of 2–6 mu/min. It is continued with geometric increases in dosage every 20–30 minutes till 4 contractions are achieved in 10 minutes (each lasting 40 seconds), with the fetal heart rate remaining normal (Table 7.1). The duration of the infusion depends mainly on the cervical response and the descent of the presenting part. At the end of 4 hours the progress is reviewed, and it could

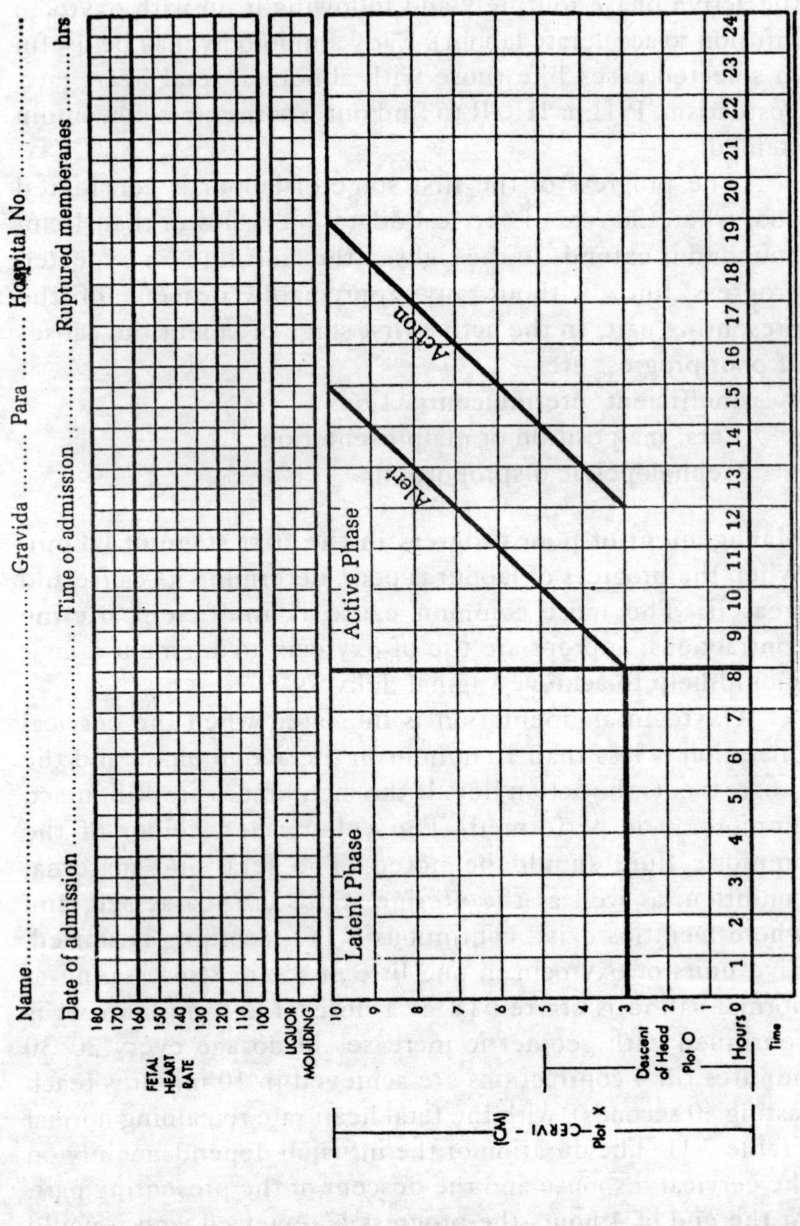

Name .... Gravida .... Para .... Hospital No. ....
Date of admission .... Time of admission .... Ruptured memberanes .... hrs
FETAL HEART RATE
180
170
160
150
140
130
120
110
100
LIQUOR
MOULDING
CERVI - (CM)
Plot X
10
9
8
7
6
5
4
3
2
1
0
Descent of Head
Plot O
Hours
Time
Latent Phase
Active Phase
Alert
Action
1
2
3
4
5
6
7
8
9
10
11
12
13
14
15
16
17
18
19
20
21
22
23
24

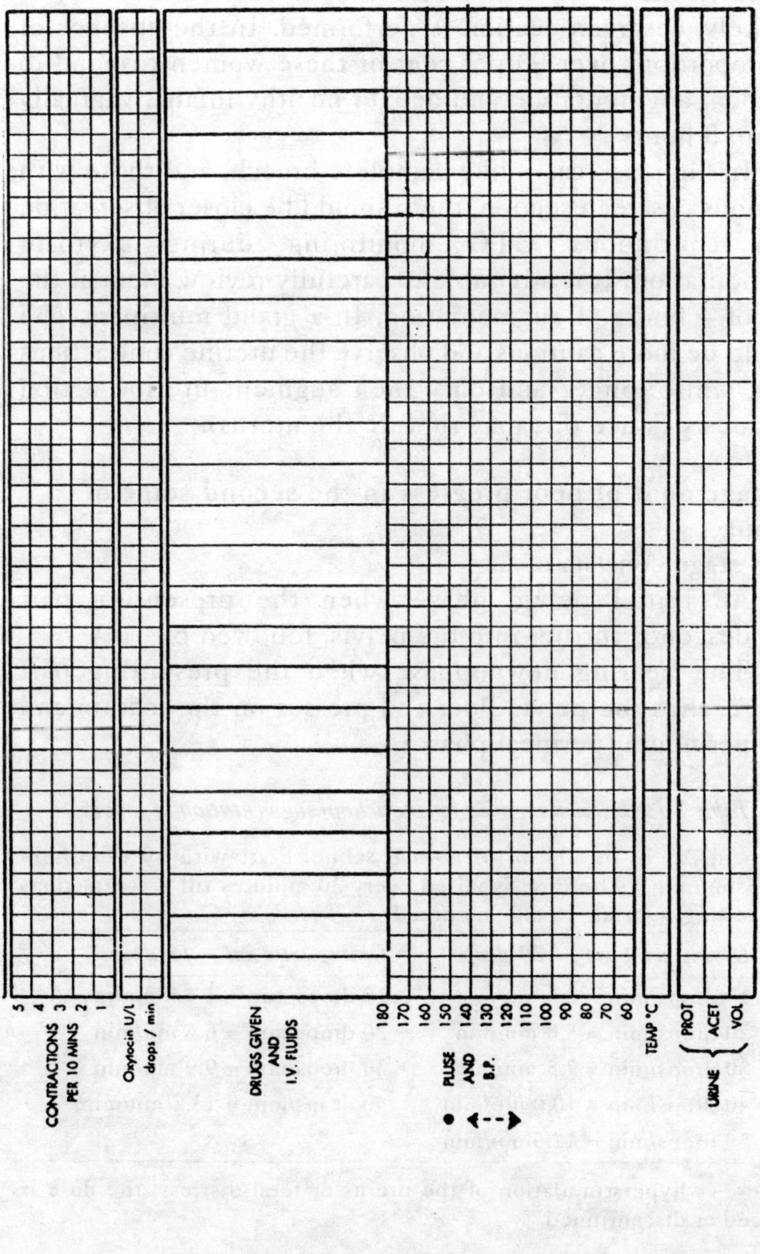

Fig 7.3 A partograph

be continued for a maximum of 4 hours more. If there is satisfactory progress, vaginal delivery is likely. If, after 8 hours, the review indicates that a vaginal delivery is unlikely, cesarean section is performed. In the absence of disproportion, over 90 per cent of these women respond to oxytocin augmentation and deliver healthy infants vaginally within 8 hours.

In high-risk cases like complete breech, and those with previous cesarean section, there should be closer observation with continuous CTG monitoring during oxytocin augmentation. It is advisable to carefully review them at the end of 4 hours of augmentation. In a grand multipara, one should be more cautious and observe the uterine contractions for a while longer and only then augment uterine action cautiously (since this may rupture the uterus).

Management of poor progress in the second stage of labour

This stage consists of

1. An initial pelvic phase when the presenting part descends further into the pelvis, followed by
2. The bearing down phase when the presenting part reaches the pelvic floor and presses on the rectum and perineum (perineal phase).

Table 7.1: Oxytocin regimen for induction/augmentation of labour

Oxytocin 2.5 iu in 500 ml of normal saline. Start with 10 drops/min (2–2.5 mu/min.) The dose is raised every 30 minutes till 4 contractions each lasting > 40 sec/10 min are noted.

Giving set 1 ml = 20 drops	*Giving set 1 ml = 15 drops*
10 drops/min = 2.5 mu/min	10 drops/min = 3.4 mu/min
20 drops/min = 5.0 mu/min	20 drops/min = 6.6 mu/min
30 drops/min = 7.5 mu/min	30 drops/min = 9.9 mu/min
40 drops/min = 10.0 mu/min	40 drops/min = 13.2 mu/min
50 drops/min = 12.5 mu/min	

If there is hyperstimulation of the uterus or fetal distress, the dose is reduced or discontinued.

It may be noted that malpresentation of the vertex (as in right occipital posterior) requires longer time and good contractions for it to reach the pelvic floor, in such cases augmentation is useful. However, in case of a large baby (as in some multiparas or in gestational diabetes with macrosomia) where there has been a protracted late first stage, any delay in the descent of the fetus at this stage should be viewed with suspicion. Augmentation or forceps application at this stage could be disastrous. It may end in a difficult high forceps, traumatic to both the mother and her child, or end in shoulder dystocia. In the second stage of labour after the head descends to the pelvic floor in case of fetal distress or delay due to maternal exhaustion, a vacuum extraction or an easy outlet forceps is carried out.

For pain relief in labour, narcotic analgesics (pethidine HCl 1 mg/kg or morphine 0.1 mg/kg) are preferred over tranquilisers like phenothiazine or diazepam. The narcotics act for 2–4 hours but, if childbirth should occur within an hour after its administration, the newborn must receive naloxone 0.02 mg IM soon after birth to prevent respiratory depression. In most modern clinics a continuous epidermal anesthesia is preferred. It gives excellent relief from pain and any operative delivery including cesarean section (if required) could be performed without additional anesthesia.

A routine episiotomy is not done for every case. It may be useful in vaginal operative deliveries as in forceps, assisted breech delivery and shoulder dystocia, in the presence of a scarred perineum, and to expedite delivery in cases of fetal distress. When the head emerges, flexion is promoted and the perineum supported. After checking for cord round the neck the anterior shoulder is delivered slowly. Simultaneously, for the active management of the third stage 0.2 mg of ergometrine is given IV (except in PIH or in cardiovascular disease where oxytocin 10 iu intravenous is preferred). Once the baby is born, check that the airway is clear, and there is no hypoxia. Apgar score at 1 and 5 minutes is noted. If the placenta has separated, it is delivered by gentle traction on the cord with simultaneous counter-traction upwards on the contracted uterus. Once the placenta is delivered and examined, ensure that the uterus remains well-contracted and retracted and there is no PPH. After checking her BP, temperature and pulse, the patient is kept warm and observed for bleeding for at least one hour.

Case Report 1

7 am: A 23-year-old primigravida was admitted with painful uterine contractions for 4 hours. She was past her due date by 5 days. On examination, she was not anemic; BP 110/70; pulse 82/min. The uterus was term size and was contracting 3/10 min, each contraction lasting for 20 seconds. The head was 1/5th felt in left occipital anterior position. The FHR was normal. Per vaginum examination revealed that the cervix was well-effaced, 4 cm dilated, head at 0 station, bag of membranes present. An ARM was done because of postdatism with escape of 200 ml clear liquor.

11 am: Painful contractions were noted at a frequency of 4/10 min each lasting for 30 seconds; head was not felt; FHR 146/min. Per vaginum examination revealed that the cervix was 8 cm dilated, membranes absent, vertex at +1, small caput but no moulding.

12.25 pm: Contractions were noted at a frequency of 4/10 min, each lasting for 40 seconds; FHR was 150/min regular; head seen on separating the labia; cervix fully dilated head at +4.

12.30 pm: Delivered a live female child; Apgar 8/10; weight 2.7 kg.

Comments: This lady had a spontaneous vaginal delivery and the progress of labour (cervical dilatation pattern) was within the alert line (Fig 7.4).

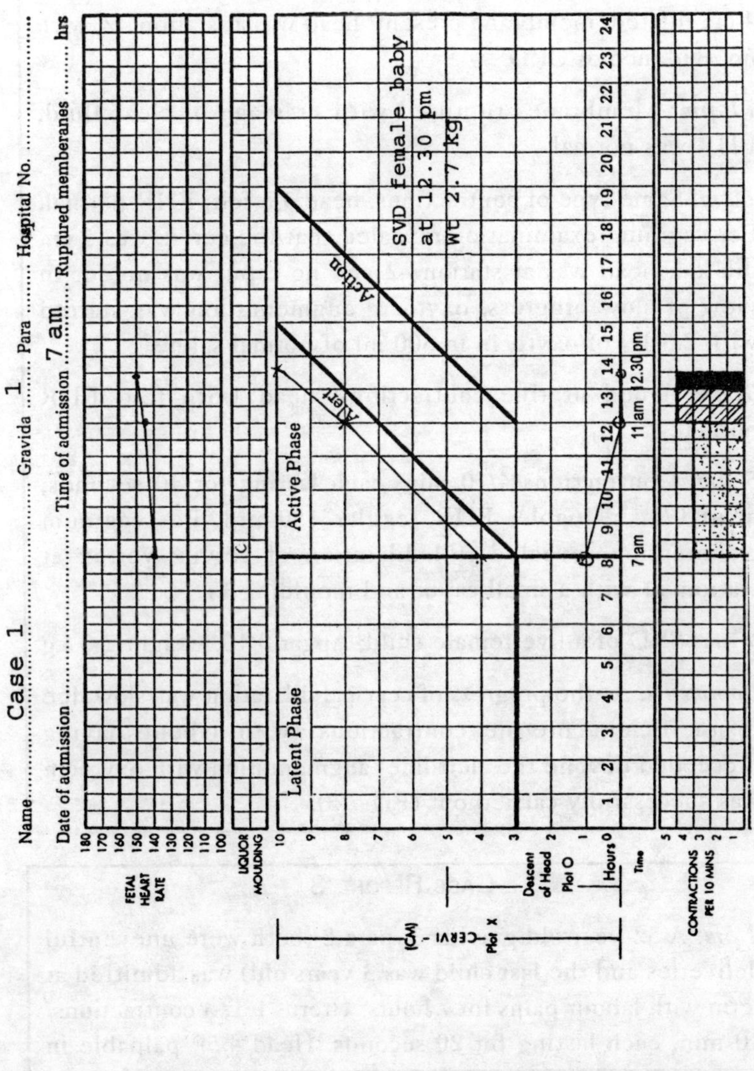

Fig 7.4 Partograph of case report 1

Case Report 2

9 pm: A 26-year-old full term pregnant woman in labour for 6 hours was admitted. The uterus was term size, contractions were 3/10 min, each lasting for 20 seconds. Head was $3/5^{th}$ palpable in LOA. FHR was 144/min. Per vaginum examination revealed that the cervix was well-effaced and 4 cm dilated; membrane present; head was at station –2, with no evidence of CPD.

11 pm: Membranes ruptured with drainage of clear fluid, FHR was normal.

1 am: Same type of contractions; head 3/5 felt; FHR normal. Per vaginum examination revealed that the cervix was 5 cm dilated; head was at station –2 and no caput was noted. In view of slow progress, oxytocin augmentation was started with 2.5 IU of oxytocin in 500 ml of normal saline.

3 am: Good uterine contractions, head 1/5th felt. FHR normal.

5 am: Contractions 4/10 min, each lasting for 40 seconds; head $0/5^{th}$ palpable; FHR regular 150/min. Per vaginum examination revealed full dilatation of cervix; vertex at station +1 with a small caput and moulding 1+.

6 am: SVD of a live female child; Apgar 8/10; weight 2.8 kg

Comments: As the progress of cervical dilatation was slow due to inefficient uterine contractions (with labour having proceeded beyond the alert line) augmentation with oxytocin was successfully carried out (Fig 7.5).

Case Report 3

3 pm: A 32-year-old gravida 3, para 2 (both were uneventful deliveries and the last child was 3 years old) was admitted at term with labour pains for 7 hours. Uterus FT, 3 contractions/ 10 min, each lasting for 20 seconds. Head $4/5^{th}$ palpable in

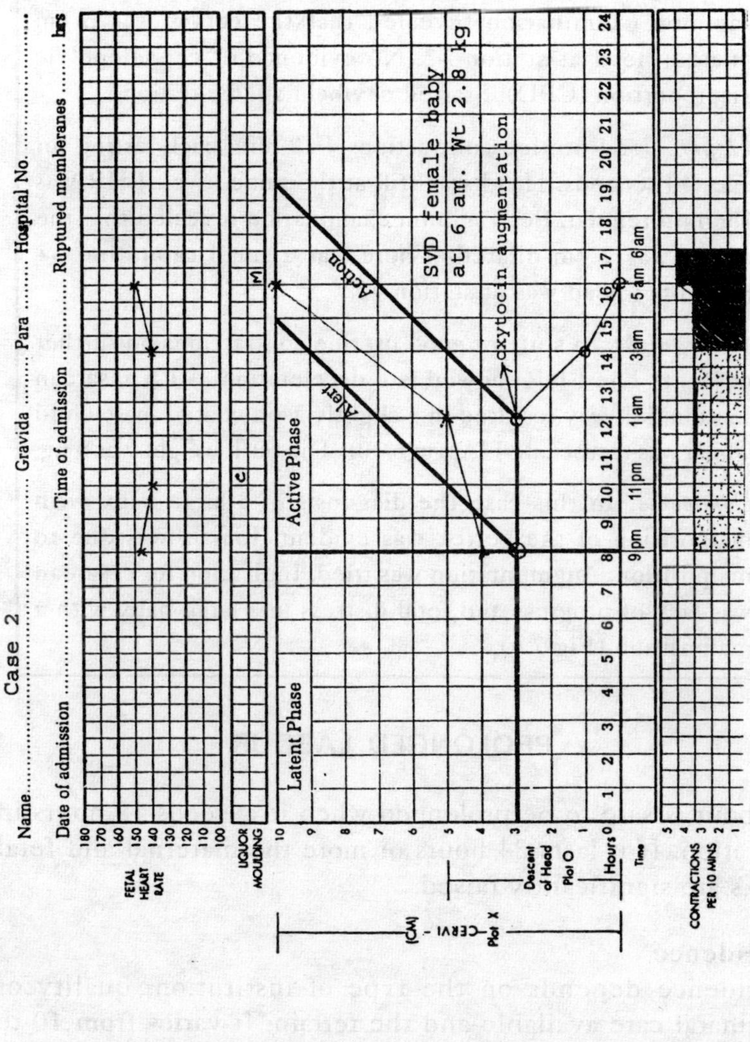

Fig 7.5 Partograph of case report 2

ROT and deflexed. FHR normal. Per vaginum examination revealed a well-effaced 5 cm dilated cervix; membranes intact but accidentally ruptured draining 150 ml of clear fluid; vertex at station –3.

7 pm: Moderate, painful contractions 3/10 min each lasting for 30 seconds; head $3/5^{th}$ felt; FHR regular 150/min. Per vaginum examination revealed that the cervix was 6 cm dilated; head at station –2. No evidence of cephalopelvic disproportion (CPD). Started oxytocin augmentation.

11 pm: Good uterine contractions 4/10 min, each lasting for over 40 seconds. Head was still at the same level. FHR was 156/min regular. Per vaginum examination revealed that the cervix was 7 cm dilated. There was a small caput and ++ moulding; head was at station –2.

12 midnight: In spite of good uterine contractions no further descent. The FHR showed late deceleration. A LS cesarean section delivery resulted in a slightly asphyxiated male child which was resuscitated (Apgar 6/10). The birth weight was 4 kg.

Comments: In this case the diagnosis of a large baby with malposition of the vertex was evident. Inertia was due to malposition. Augmentation was tried. Indication for cesarean was lack of progress and fetal distress in a large baby with a malposition (Fig 7.6).

PROLONGED LABOUR

Labour is said to be prolonged when it exceeds 18 hours in duration. If it lasts 24 hours or more the maternal and fetal risks are significantly raised.

Incidence

Incidence depends on the type of institution, quality of perinatal care available and the terrain. It varies from 10 to 20 per cent in developing countries.

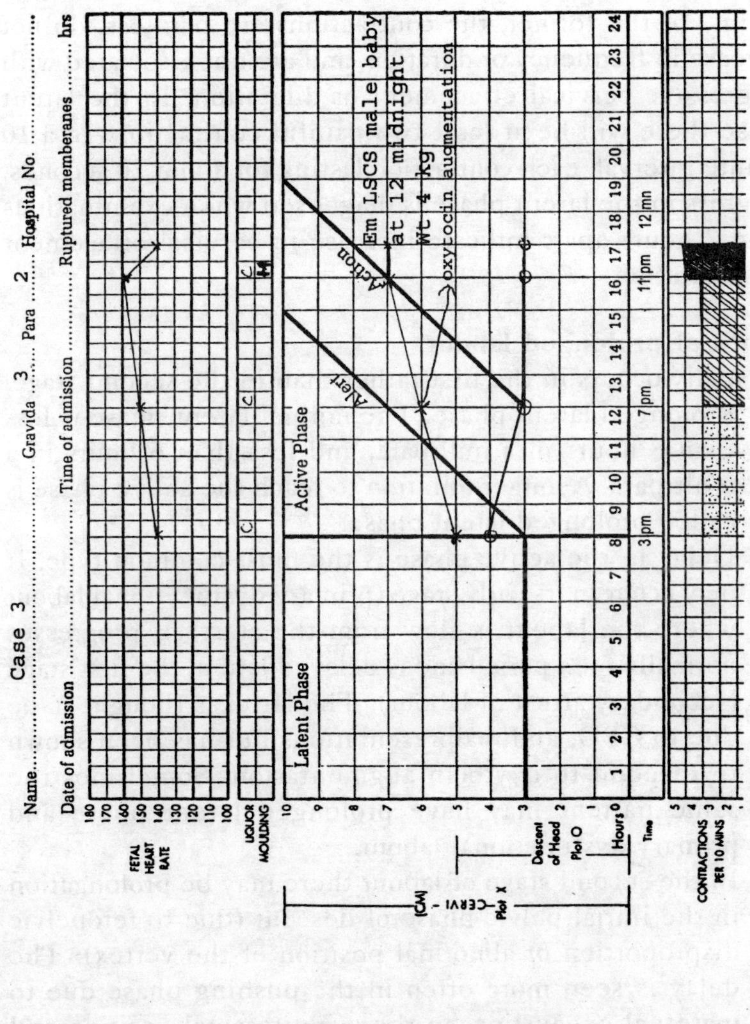

Fig 7.6 Partograph of case report 3

Etiology

In over 70 per cent of cases prolonged labour is due to inefficient uterine contractions. Other causes are cephalopelvic disproportion (CPD), malpresentations and malpositions like occipitoposterior position of vertex.

The endpoint of labour is well-defined, but not its beginning. False labour must be distinguished from true labour. In the former, the contractions are painless, do not increase in frequency or duration, and are not associated with progressive cervical effacement or dilatation. In the latent phase there will be at least two painful contractions in a 10 minute interval, each contraction lasting for about 20 seconds. Progress in the latent phase is diagnosed when examinations done 2 hours apart indicate increase in cervical effacement and dilatation.

Types of prolonged labour

It usually occurs in the first rather than in the second stage.

1. Prolonged latent phase. The normal latent phase is less than 8 hours in a nullipara, and less than 6 hours in a multipara. A longer duration to reach the active phase is called prolonged latent phase.
2. Delay in the active phase is the most common type. It may occur in its early stage (primary dysfunctional labour where the labour is slow from the start) or progresses normally for a period and is delayed late in the first stage (secondary arrest of labour). The latter is thought to be due to CPD, and malpresentations but has been shown to respond to oxytocin augmentation. Sometimes the same patient may have prolonged latent phase and primary dysfunctional labour.
3. In the second stage of labour there may be prolongation in the initial pelvic phase of descent (due to fetopelvic disproportion or abnormal position of the vertex). The delay is seen more often in the pushing phase due to maternal exhaustion, in the occipitosacral position and

face to pubis delivery, or in those under epidural anesthesia.

4. When labour is prolonged, often in the neglected second stage, and further descent of the fetus is arrested due to mechanical factors, labour is said to be 'obstructed'. In such cases, spontaneous delivery is impossible and unless professional help is immediately available to deliver the baby, it will end in rupture of the uterus. This type of prolonged labour is the most dangerous but is entirely preventable. Good perinatal care, partographic recording during labour to help identify abnormal labour and appropriate action, should reduce the incidence of prolonged labour.

Diagnosis of prolonged labour is made when labour exceeds 18 hours. Except in those in the second stage when the uterus may be contracting well to overcome deflexion of the head or obstruction in the pelvis, uterine contractions are usually sluggish in other cases. The partograph (Fig 7.6) shows that the action line has been crossed and appropriate action has not been taken.

Complications

Maternal complications

Prolonged labour leads to dehydration and ketosis. After rupture of the membranes it may cause chorioamnionitis, increased operative delivery rates, PPH, puerperal sepsis and PID. In obstructed labour the risks to the mother are greater.

Fetal complications

For the fetus, there is increased perinatal hypoxia, infection, intracranial injury, convulsions, delayed milestones, cerebral palsy and increased perinatal mortality.

Management

Preventive measures are good prenatal screening, use of partography and timely interventions as indicated.

1. In the prolonged latent phase, after ruling out CPD,

hypoxia and malpresentations, assurance, rehydration, ambulation and pain relief are indicated. If oxytocin augmentation is tried at this phase there is a risk of fetal distress due to increased uterine activity. This might lead to an unnecessary cesarean section.

2. In the early active phase of labour, if the delay is due to inefficient contractions causing inadequate cervical dilatation that crosses the action line, one has to first rule out CPD and malpresentations before carrying out oxytocin augmentation. In case of CPD and abnormal presentations with thick, loosely applied cervix, a cesarean section is indicated. It is also necessary in the few patients who do not progress in response to oxytocin augmentation, and in those with evidence of fetal distress.
3. In the delayed second stage, if there is no descent in spite of good contractions fetopelvic disproportion may be the cause and a cesarean section is indicated. In occipitoposterior presentation, the delay is due to wrong internal rotation. If the general condition of mother and fetus are satisfactory, and contractions are not good (less than 4 contractions in 1 minute, each lasting less than 40 seconds), a carefully monitored oxytocin infusion is started. If the patient responds, she may spontaneously deliver vaginally or with forceps. If there is no progress a cesarean section is performed.
4. In case of delay at the pelvic floor, the delivery is achieved with vacuum or outlet forceps, provided the lowest part of the head (and not the caput) is well below the level of the ischial spines.

In all cases of prolonged active phase of labour:

- Dextrose saline IV is maintained to prevent dehydration and ketosis.
- Prophylactic oxytocics are necessary after the birth of the anterior shoulder, to prevent PPH.

OBSTRUCTED LABOUR

In obstructed labour, the labour is at a standstill with the presenting part jammed in the pelvis due to mechanical factors, with no chance of a spontaneous delivery.

Incidence

The incidence is about 1–5 per cent of deliveries depending on the standard of health care and transport facilities available to the community.

Etiology

It results from neglected labour. The important causes are:

1. Cephalopelvic disproportion (CPD)
2. Malpresentations: shoulder or face (mentoposterior)
3. Malposition as in occipitoposterior,
4. Fetal anomalies: hydrocephalus (rare)
5. Soft tissue obstructions: scarred cervix, myoma or large stone in the bladder (Rao 1996)

Signs, symptoms and diagnosis

The diagnosis is made from history of prolonged labour of over 18 hours, and after 3–4 hours have passed since the rupture of membranes. The patient looks exhausted, dehydrated, often infected with slight pyrexia and tachycardia. The upper part of the uterus looks markedly contracted and retracted, lower uterine segment well—stretched out and tender with a transverse ring about the level of umbilicus (Bandl's ring, Fig 7.7). The presenting part is jammed in the pelvis and the fetal heart rate is either irregular, rapid or absent. Per vaginum: a fully dilated cervix, with marked moulding and huge caput over the presenting part which fills up the congested vagina. (In a neglected shoulder it may be the edematous prolapsed hand.) Offensive vaginal discharge may be present in some cases.

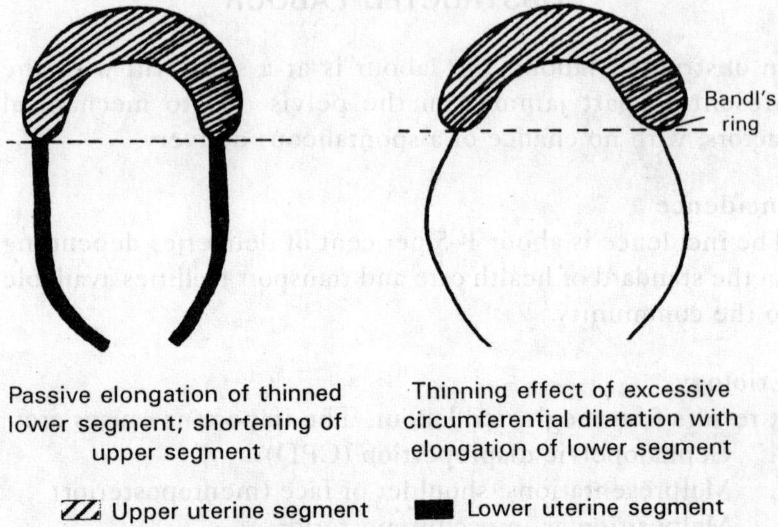

Fig 7.7 Changes in the upper and lower uterine segments in obstructed labour

The examination often helps to find out the cause of the obstruction, integrity of the uterus, condition of the fetus and the station of the presenting part. Catheterisation usually shows blood stained urine.

Prognosis

Maternal mortality is about 3–5 per cent. Perinatal mortality is quite high (about 75 per cent) due to anoxia, trauma and sepsis.

Maternal complications are ruptured uterus in 10–15 per cent, PPH and puerperal sepsis. Among the sequelae are vesicovaginal fistula due to ischemic necrosis in 1–5 per cent and in some, peroneal palsy may also be seen.

Management

Preventive

Good prenatal and intranatal care including partography.

Curative

1. Correct rehydration by rapid administration of IV fluids:

1 litre of normal saline or Ringer lactate solution.

2. Combat sepsis with parenteral broad spectum antibiotics ampicillin 500 mg 6 hourly and metronidazole 500 mg 8 hourly IV. Keep 1 unit of compatible blood ready.
3. Under general anesthesia, empty the uterus without stretching or distending it further (No IP version).

Fetus alive

- Head engaged with 1/5th or less palpable. Vaginally easy instrumental delivery if possible. The baby will need to be resuscitated and treated for intranatal infection.
- Head unengaged or malpresentation: cesarean section.

Fetus dead

- Fully dilated cervix and unengaged head: Craniotomy if one has experience; if not CS (chapter 10)
- Hydrocephalus: Ask an assistant to fix the head suprapubically. With the help of a perforator or a sharp pointed scissors perforate the head (through cervix that is reasonably dilated to safely carry out the procedure) and after letting out the cerebrospinal fluid allow the patient rest. The decompressed head and fetus will easily be born vaginally.
- Hand prolapse: Neglected shoulder presentation: decapitation is the treatment of choice (chapter 10).

If the physician is not experienced or trained in destructive procedures, cesarean section has to be performed.

In all cases of obstructed labour after emptying the uterus, remove the placenta manually and explore the uterus to ensure there is no rupture. Prevent PPH with oxytocin and sepsis with antibiotics. Drain the bladder for a week to prevent bladder fistula.

RUPTURE OF THE UTERUS

Rupture of the uterus is one of the most serious obstetric emergencies and accounts for 5–10 per cent of maternal deaths in developing countries.

Incidence

Incidence is about 1 in 1000 deliveries, but in a referral hospital and in peripheral areas where rapid transport services are not available, it is higher.

Etiology

It is more common in labour than in pregnancy. In pregnancy uterine rupture may be due to weakness in the myometrium as in pregnancy following a classic cesarean section, myomectomy (post-laparoscopic) or a vigorous curettage.

During labour, rupture of the uterus may be

1. Spontaneous, as a result of neglected or obstructed labour, commonly reported in developing countries
2. Rupture of the lower uterine segment cesarean scar (common in developed regions)
3. Traumatic, for example, following IP version, late in labour, forceps or breech extractions through an incompletely dilated cervix and due to injudicious administration of oxytocics for induction or augmentation.

Diagnosis

The patient may give previous history of uterine surgery or history of prolonged labour, or an operative delivery.

CASE REPORT 4

1 pm: A 33-year-old unbooked gravida 4, para 3 (with previous normal deliveries), was admitted with history of labour since 9 pm previous day. The contractions were mild initially, but after rupture of membranes at 6 am, she had strong contractions for 3 hours after which the painful contractions stopped. On the advice of her untrained attendant she sought admission.

On examination, she appeared exhausted and pale; pulse 120/min, BP 90/?. Per abdomen: fetal parts were felt very superficially; the uterine outline was lost. Per vaginum: cervix fully dilated head jammed in pelvis at station –2 with a large caput. She was started on IV normal saline and Ringer lactate (500 ml each) at a rapid rate. Two units of cross—matched blood were immediately obtained from the blood bank. Prophylactic antibiotics (ampicillin 500 mg and metronidazole 0.5 g) were given IV (chapter 18). On emergency laparotomy, uterus was found to have ruptured anteriorly with a dead fetus (female, 4 kg) and placenta in peritoneal cavity along with free blood and clots, after removal of which the lower segment rent was repaired along with ligation of the tubes. The abdomen was closed.

She received 2 units of blood during the operation. General condition at the end of the procedure was satisfactory, BP 100/70, pulse 110/min. For the next 48 hours IV fluids and antibiotics were given till oral feeds and medications were started on 3rd postoperative day and she was discharged on 8th postoperative day with advice to continue oral iron for the next 8 weeks.

Case Report 5

8 am: A 27-year-old booked gravida 2, para 1, who had a LS cesarean delivery 3 years earlier (for fetal distress and unengaged head in late 1 stage; live male 2.8 kg alive now) was admitted at 8 am, an hour after the painful contractions started (2 days prior to her EDD). She had been assessed earlier for a trial of vaginal delivery.

On examination, uterus was term, contractions 3/10 min, each lasting for 20 seconds. Head was well flexed; 4/5 felt per abdomen LOA; FHR was normal.

Per vaginum: Cervix centrally placed almost fully effaced and 2 cm dilated. Bag of membranes were felt and the head was at station –3. No evidence of CPD.

10 am: Membranes ruptured and clear fluid was seen. FHR was normal. She was put on continuous monitoring with CTG.

12 noon: Contractions 4 per 10 min, each lasted for 30–40 seconds, head 2/5th felt; FHR regular 140–146/min. PV cervix 6 cm membranes absent, vertex was at –1 with no moulding.

12:23 pm: Same abdominal findings as before except that the FH is slow now at 100/min (maternal pulse 110/min) and there was slight suprapubic tenderness. Emergency cesarean section was done. There was dehiscence of the scar. The child was delivered through it and revived (Apgar 5/10 at 1 minute and 9/10 at 5 minutes; weight 2.7 kg). After delivering the placenta, the rent in the lower segment was closed and was followed by tubal sterilisation. At the end of the operation, maternal condition was good. BP 120/80 mmHg, pulse 104 /min. Postoperative period was uneventful. Mother and child were discharged on the 8th postoperative day.

Comments on cases 4 and 5: Case 4 is a typical example of a spontaneous complete rupture as a result of neglected obstetrics. She had strong contractions for 3 hours (after the membranes ruptured or in the second stage) trying to push down a big baby, which was in a malposition. She reached a stage of threatened rupture and when no help came the overstretched LU segment gave way with escape of fetus and placenta through the rent and the uterus ceased to act. When she reported in a stage of shock, uterine contour was lost and fetus was felt superficially. As the rent was fairly clean it was repaired and to prevent recurrence, she was sterilised. She had antiprolactins to suppress lactation.

In this patient, hysterectomy would have added to the shock. In a case of rupture, hysterectomy is needed if the rent is

- Irregular, friable and infected
- In a lateral uterine wall rupture where the uterine artery (mostly left) is torn producing a broad ligament hematoma

- In colporrhexis, where rupture involves the vaginal fornix.

In case 5, the risk of rupture of a previous LSCS scar in a subsequent labour is about 1 per cent. A case is chosen for a trial of vaginal delivery after considering all details of previous surgery and ruling out CPD, malpresentations etc. She has to be monitored carefully in an institution where the theatre, obstetricians and anesthetist are readily available so that at the earliest evidence of impending scar dehiscence or fetal distress cesarean section could be performed. In this case fetal heart rate abnormalities, maternal tachycardia and suprapubic tenderness helped to detect the rupture early. This is an atypical type as the fetus is still in utero. The prognosis for mother and child are largely good in scar dehiscence. It is worst in traumatic rupture as the diagnosis is delayed or missed after an operative delivery.

Another atypical variety of rupture is seen in spontaneous type with a broad ligament hematoma (Fig 7.8). In this type, which clinically resembles abruptio placentae, there is tenderness and fullness, mostly on the left side, slight vaginal bleeding, tachycardia with slow or absent FH sounds. As the uterine outline is still present (with the fetus still in utero) the delay in diagnosis worsens the prognosis. This type of rupture requires a hysterectomy and ligation of the retracted severed end of the uterine artery.

Prognosis

In a rupture of the uterus prognosis is best in LSCS scar rupture (maternal < 1 per cent and perinatal < 10 per cent) compared to the other two types where maternal mortality is 5–8 per cent and PMR 35–50 per cent.

Note

- Do not extract a baby through an incompletely dilated cervix.

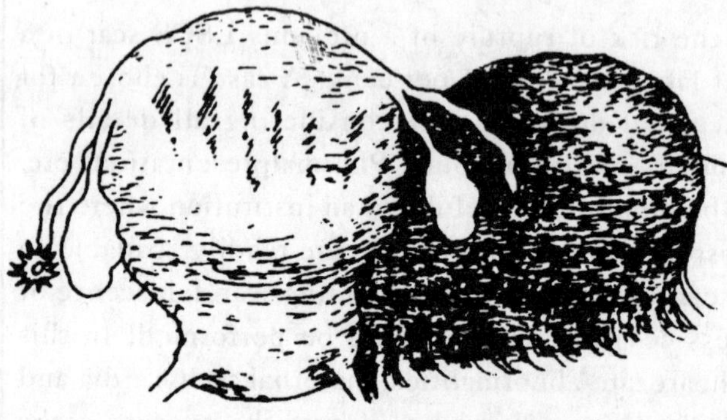

Fig 7.8 Rupture uterus

- Do not delay 2nd stage in a woman with a uterine scar.
- Do not do a destructive operation unless you are trained and experienced in doing it.
- Do not do an IP version in a case of previous cesarean or in a case of late labour.
- Do not use misoprostol for induction of labour in a case of previous cesarean section.
- Do not persist in doing a manual removal of a placenta where no plane of cleavage is found. Forcible attempts may end in perforation of uterus and bleeding.
- Do not attempt vaginal delivery in a case of suspected uterine rupture. You may widen the rent and the postpartum collapse may delay diagnosis and worsen the prognosis.

FETAL DISTRESS

A healthy fetus in utero is normally active as made out by its movements and baseline variability of its heart rate. But under conditions of hypoxia, fetal distress is indicated by reduction in its movements and slowing of its cardiac activity. When the hypoxia is acute and prolonged, all its activity ceases and it dies.

Incidence

Incidence is about 5–8 per cent.

Etiology

Fetal distress results from hypoxia or reduced oxygen supply to its tissues especially to the vital organs, heart and brain. The hypoxia may be intermittent, acute or chronic (prolonged). It may be seen:

1. Antepartum: In placental insufficiency, IUGR, PIH, abruptio placentae, diabetes, thrombophilia and prolonged pregnancy.
2. Intrapartum: All of the above causes, in CPD, due to excessive moulding in prolonged or obstructed labour (due to prolonged period of contractions), hypertonic uterus or cord prolapse
3. Neonatal: In a depressed (sedated) or hypoxoic baby. This is indicated by Apgar scoring and pulmonary or neurological sequelae of hypoxia.

Signs, symptoms and diagnosis

Fetal activity requires oxygen and glucose. The fetus responds to hypoxia by reducing its active movements. There may be compensatory tachycardia in a gradually developing hypoxia while the fetus slows down its heart rate in acute hypoxia due to vagal stimulation. At times it relaxes the anal sphincter with escape of thick meconium into liquor amnii. In case of fetal tachycardia, rule out maternal fever, tocolytic drugs and chorioamnionitis before concluding that it is due to fetal distress.

In the antepartum period: The assessment of fetal compromise can be made by

- Palpation and measurement of fundal height

- Kick count or number of fetal movements felt by the mother during a known interval; 4 in 2 hours or 10 in 12 hours
- Doppler flow velocimetry of the umbilical and middle cerebral arteries (MCA)
- Reactivity to non-stress test (NST)
- By USG study of fetal muscle tone, number of respiratory and active limb movements, amount of liquor amnii as measured by amniotic fluid index (biophysical profile).

The liquor volume varies depending on fetal well-being. The volume of liquor is the balance of that swallowed and of urine passed by the fetus. The normal AFI is 10; if it is less than 5 there is possible fetal compromise; if it is below 2 there is impending fetal demise. Each of these four parameters and NST which constitute the biophysical profile (BPP) carry 2 points and a score of 10 indicates the fetus is healthy; below 6 indicates possible fetal compromise.

Early diagnosis of intrapartum fetal distress is important. This is done by:

- Monitoring fetal heart rate (FHR) either by intermittent auscultation (every 15 minutes in the first stage and at 5 minute intervals in the second stage) or by continuous electronic fetal monitoring (EFM) with CTG, which is more sensitive to detect loss of baseline variability. It will also show loss of accelerations, late deceleration caused by hypoxia due to inadequate placental circulation or variable deceleration due to cord compression. However, as its specificity is low and to avoid unnecessary cesarean sections other methods are also used in addition to refine its diagnostic accuracy.
- As hypoxia leads to increased accumulation of CO_2 or lactate in the tissues, pH estimation of fetal scalp blood (FSB) (for metabolic acidosis) or of lactate by micromethods have been found to be useful.

- Other methods used for detection of fetal distress are fetal oximetry to measure SO_2 and fetal ECG recordings
- Presence of thick meconium except in breech is a clinically useful indicator of possible fetal distress.

Diagnosis of neonatal hypoxia is usually obvious because the child does not breathe or cry at birth. The Apgar score depends on observation of five signs—heart rate, respiratory effort, reflex irritability, muscle tone and colour. A score of 0, 1 and 2 is given to each sign: 0 indicates absence of the sign. A total of 10 points indicate that the baby is in the best possible condition. The score at 1 minute appraises the need for resuscitation and the score at 5 minutes is probable predictor of late neurodevelopmental disability. However, it should be emphasised that there is no neonatal parameter at birth that can accurately predict neurodevelopmental disability. Most babies who survive with low Apgar scores do not develop cerebral palsy. It is now concluded that a diagnosis of encephalopathy due to perinatal hypoxia requires evidence of neonatal neurological abnormalities and multiorgan dysfunction in addition to a low 5 minute Apgar score along with neonatal acidosis. However, there are reports to show that a 5 minute score of below 3 is indicative of a severely compromised infant with a poor chance of survival.

Prognosis

Prognosis depends on the duration and intensity of hypoxia, the period of gestation and the associated etiological factors. It is believed that cerebral palsy may result not so much due to intrapartum or neonatal hypoxia but usually follows intermittent prolonged (chronic) hypoxia. If the hypoxia is acute and prolonged, the fetus dies in utero. With a 5 minute Apgar score of 3 or less, neonatal death is a probability. Meconium aspiration syndrome has poor prognosis. Complications of fetal distress in a premature infant include pulmonary complications, cerebral intraventricular hemorrhages, convulsions and neurodevelopmental defects.

Management of fetal distress

Preventive: Good prenatal care and careful intrapartum monitoring with partography, and avoidance of injudicious use of oxytocics.

Detection: Fundal height measurements, kick counts, Doppler flowmetry and BPP have been described earlier along with their critical values indicative of fetal distress.

- Cesarean section is indicated in cases of abruptio placentae. In cases of severe IUGR or PIH when the Doppler flow of the umbilical artery or MCA is unsatisfactory, a careful decision needs to be made for induction or cesarean section.
- After 37 weeks, at the earliest evidence of fetal distress, the child could be delivered depending on the cervical score. If the hypoxia is acute, delivery is by immediate cesarean section. When labour is induced continuous EFM is necessary. Early amniotomy may show thick meconium with scanty fluid. When hypoxia is suspected emergency CS should be done.
- The decision is difficult between 26 and 32 weeks in view of the high PMR in immature VLBW babies. In institutions with neonatal intensive care units (NICU), the cesarean section is done in consultation with the neonatologist.
- Between 32 and 37 weeks if cesarean section is needed, it is best done after betamethasone administration to promote pulmonary maturity.
- When intrapartum hypoxia is suspected with EFM, if facilities are available pH of fetal scalp blood is estimated to confirm acidosis (pH < 7.20) prior to cesarean section. When the cervix is fully dilated and the head is 1/5 or less palpable, forceps delivery could be attempted. In cord prolapse, when it is pulsating, postural manual replacement into the vagina should be followed by emergency cesarean section. In the presence of thick

meconium stained liquor if the cervix is fully dilated and the head is 1/5 to 0/5 palpable, instrumental vaginal delivery can be performed. If not, a cesarean section should be considered.

- Management of neonatal hypoxia is discussed in chapter 14.

MALPRESENTATIONS

When the presenting part of the fetus in the pelvis is other than vertex presentation, the presentation is called a malpresentation. Breech, shoulder, face and brow presentations are considered malpresentations; they carry increased risks for the mother and her child.

Incidence

Breech presentations are seen in about 3 per cent; shoulder and face (with brow) form 0.5 per cent each. Thus, about 4 per cent of all deliveries are malpresentations.

Etiology

Important causes are:

1. Contracted pelvis
2. Uterine anomalies
3. Fetal anomalies like anencephaly (face) and hydrocephalus (breech)
4. Placenta previa and tumours at the pelvic brim.

Face presentation

Diagnosis is suspected when on palpation the fetal cephalic pole at the pelvis consists mainly of the occiput separating it from the back by a groove due to the marked extension of the head, the sinciput not being palpable. This can be confirmed by ultrasonography and vaginal examination especially after rupture of membranes when mentum, chin, mouth and lips could be felt.

Management

In the absence of CPD a vaginal delivery could be expected in mentoanterior positions. In mentoposterior position if the chin fails to rotate in spite of good pains cesarean section is needed. In face presentations if there is a delay in the second stage of labour forceps may be applied only after the chin has reached the pelvic floor and rotated anteriorly. It must be remembered that unlike in vertex when the chin is at level of ischial spines the biparietal diameter is still well above the pelvic brim.

BROW PRESENTATION

Brow presentation is rare and is intermediate between fully flexed vertex and fully extended face presentations. In brow presentation, cesarean section is the only way to deliver (as the engaging submento-bregmatic diameter (13.5 cm) is greater than any pelvic diameters).

TRANSVERSE LIE – SHOULDER PRESENTATION

Diagnosis

It can be diagnosed with ease as in this case the transverse axis of the uterus is more than the longitudinal axis with the fetal head felt in one of the flanks. In an oblique lie, the head or breech may be palpable in either of the iliac fossas and the breech or head in the opposite hypochondrium. The fetal heart is heard on the same plane as the umbilicus.

Management

Though a small premature baby may be born doubled up spontaneously, there is little chance of a spontaneous vaginal delivery after 30 weeks.

1. In the absence of an obvious cause like placenta previa, contracted pelvis or tumours (where CS is indicated), an external cephalic version (ECV) is tried at 32–34 weeks or even at term when transverse lie is seen.

2. If it fails, elective cesarean section is indicated.
3. If she is admitted in labour as a transverse lie with a good fetal heart rate an emergency cesarean section is performed if the ECV fails.
4. If she is admitted soon after rupture of membranes with uterus completely relaxed between contractions and the cervix is fully dilated IP version and extraction can be tried as an alternative to cesarean section. However, caution should be exercised because of the possibility of uterine rupture.
5. At the time of admission if there is hand and cord prolapse with no cord pulsations, IP version is done and the foot is brought down if the cervix is not fully dilated. Breech is delivered later after full dilatation to avoid traumatic PPH. In such a case if the fetus were alive an emergency cesarean section should be done.
6. In a neglected shoulder presentation with a dead fetus the choice is between decapitation and a cesarean section depending on the experience of the physician (chapters 8 and 10).

Breech presentation

Breech presentation is a reversal of normal polarity, with the fetal head at the fundus and the podalic pole at the pelvic brim. Three types of breech presentations are known:

1. Complete or flexed breech maintaining the attitude of universal flexion including at the hip and knee
2. Extended breech seen mostly in primiparas, with legs flexed at the hip but extended at the knees. The breech is fixed at the pelvic brim and the feet at the fundus covering the face.
3. Breech with knee or footling presentation.

Diagnosis

Mapping out the complete breech is easy as one could easily feel the firm ballottable head at the fundus, and a soft broad breech floating at the pelvic brim with the fetal heart being audible above the umbilicus usually on the left and anteriorly (left sacroanterior (LSA) being the commonest position).

The extended breech however is often missed because the fetal head at the fundus is covered by the feet and it is not easily ballottable. Besides, as the breech here is well-fixed in the pelvis and the fetal heart is audible below the level of the umbilicus, a mistaken diagnosis of vertex with engaged head is often made. The mistake is discovered only after a pelvic examination or following ultrasonography. The knee and footling presentation is detected after a pelvic examination or on ultrasonography. In all cases of uncomplicated breech an ultrasonography is useful near term to rule out any fetal anomaly, estimate fetal weight, locate placental site and to confirm the type of breech and its position prior to its further management.

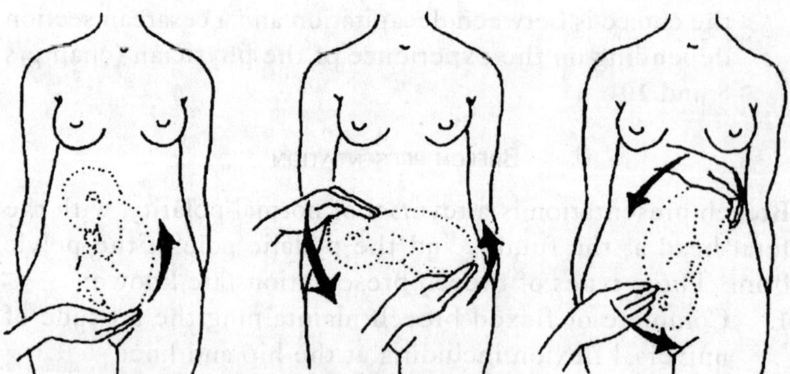

A. Mobilisation of breech

B. Manual forward rotation using both hands, one to push the breech and the other to guide the vertex

C. Completion of forward roll

Fig 7.9 External version of a breech presentation

Management

As breech is a malpresentation with higher perinatal risks, ECV is advised in all cases of uncomplicated breech ideally between 34–36 weeks (Fig 7.9). It could be attempted near the EDD or even in the early first stage of labour. It is safer if done under ultrasonographic guidance after explaining the procedure to the patient. Tocolytics are used if necessary. The fetus is turned slowly over a period of at least 15–20 minutes (fetal heart being checked often) by maintaining the attitude of flexion. Contraindications for ECV are HDP, APH, CPD and elderly primipara. If she is Rh negative, she is given prophylactic immunisation. The overall success rate of ECV is about 65–70 per cent and chances of turning back to breech are fewer in extended breech presentation.

In those breech cases where the ECV has failed the choice is between elective cesarean section at 38 weeks or a trial of vaginal breech delivery. Currently the trend is in favour of CS as it gives the child a better chance of survival and less morbidity. However, one should also realise that an abdominal delivery has 5–7 times higher risk of maternal mortality than a vaginal delivery, in addition to the risks of repeat cesarean section or scar rupture in a subsequent delivery. A child born by cesarean section is also not completely free of the risk of morbidity. Thus a balanced view at present especially in developing countries is for cesarean section in selected cases like CPD, HDP, APH, BOH footling presentations, hyperextended head (star-gazing breech) and for fetal weight above 3.5 kg. The others could be offered a trial of vaginal breech delivery. In those allowed a trial if there is lack of progress in spite of good contractions or fetal distress an emergency cesarean section is indicated. In cases of hydrocephalus, vaginal delivery is allowed after tapping the head per abdomen or after a spinal tap. Vaginal breech delivery is described in chapter 10.

Bibliography

Arulkumaran S 1999. Management of spontaneous labour. In SS Ratnam et al (Eds) *Obstetrics and Gynecology for Postgraduates*. Vol. 1, 2nd edn. 109–123.

Arulkumaran S and **Chua S** 1994. Augmentation in labour. In SS Ratnam, DK Sen et al (Eds) *Contributions to OBGYN*. Vol 3. New Delhi: BI Churchill, 175–177.

Halmesmaki E 2001. Vaginal term breech delivery – a time for reappraisal? *Acta Obstet Gynecol Scand* 80: 187–190.

Hannah M, Hannah W, Hewson SA et al 2000. Planned cesarean section vs planned vaginal birth at term: a randomised multicentre trial. *Lancet* 356: 1375.

Kamala J 1995. Obstructed labour: review of 126 cases. *J Obstet Gynecol Ind* 49: 57–59.

Mukhopadhyay S and **Arulkumaran S** 2003. Perinatal hypoxia. In SS Ratnam, Rao KB and S Arulkumaran (Eds) *Obstetrics and Gynecology for Postgraduates*. Vol 2, 2nd edn. Chennai: Orient Longman.

Papile I 2001. The Apgar Score in the 21st century. *N Engl J Med* 344: 519–20.

Rao KB 1996. Prolonged labour. In S Arulkumaran et al (Eds) *Management of Labour*. Chennai: Orient Longman.

Sadovsky E 1985. Monitoring fetal movements – a useful screening test. *Curr Obstet Gynecol* 25: 123–27.

Stronge JM 1994. Strategies for reduction of CS rates. In DR Popkins and KJ Peble (Eds) *Women's Health Today*. London: Parthenon, 55–58.

WHO 1994. Partographic management of labour. *Lancet* 343: 1399–1404.

8. Multiple pregnancy

A pregnancy in which more than one fetus is in utero is defined as a multiple pregnancy. It is a high-risk condition and carries a risk higher than in a singleton pregnancy both to the mother and to her fetuses.

Incidence

Incidence varies from 1 in 80 to 1 in 150 deliveries. The incidence of monozygotic twins, the world over, is fairly constant at 4–5 per 1000, but for dizygotic ones it varies from 4 to 50 per 1000. The latter have shown a rise of 20–30 per cent in some countries in the past decade.

Etiology

Monozygotic twins arise from a single fertilised ovum when it divides into two and each grows into a separate fetus (so-called 'identical twins'). Dizygotic twins are formed by fertilisation of two separate ova. As polyovulation occurs in certain families, these twins are familial. With assisted reproductive techniques such as in vitro fertilisation (IVF) and embryo transfer (ET), when superovulation occurs, one may find triplets to septuplets. But as 'two is company and three a crowd' the more the number of fetuses, the earlier is the termination of pregnancy. In monozygotic twins when the fertilised ovum separates late but incompletely, conjoint twins result.

Diagnosis

When i) the uterus is disproportionately enlarged for the period of amenorrhea, ii) on palpation, too many fetal small parts are felt and iii) the fetal heart is best heard in two different places on auscultation with the Doppler, one should suspect twins. Occasionally, one may feel one small head or two small heads (multiple poles) or malpresentations.

In all cases of multiple pregnancies the ultrasonography is most useful, not only to confirm the number of fetuses and their zygosity but also to check for hydramnios, fetal anomalies and malpresentations, if any. In twins, both fetuses presenting as vertex is the commonest presentation followed by one vertex and breech, or both presenting as breech; both presenting as transverse lie is the least common presentation.

Complications

Maternal complications: The chances of PIH, hydramnios, APH, anemia, malpresentations, uterine inertia and PPH are increased two–or threefold in a multiple pregnancy. Fetal prematurity, IUGR, fetal anomaly, hypoxia and perinatal mortality are increased, depending on the period of gestation and the zygosity.

The perinatal mortality is about 2–3 times the rate reported in singletons. It varies with:

1. Birth weight
2. Period of gestation at birth
3. Associated complications
4. It is slightly increased in the second of twins
5. It is slightly increased in monozygous twins: it is the worst in monochorionic monoamniotic type. Monochorionic twins may also show evidence of feto-fetal transfusion due to their vascular anastomoses in the placenta. As a result, one of them may die early and is compressed (fetus papyraceous) or malformed (acardiac and amorphic), anemic or retained in utero after its demise, threatening the survival of the other.

Management

During pregnancy

1. Advice is given about rest, exercise, nutrition, oral iron and folates to prevent anemia.
2. In the second and last trimesters she is monitored carefully to see whether she develops any of the complications mentioned earlier. If present, treat her for it at the earliest.
3. Ultrasonography is performed at 20 weeks to rule out fetal anomalies and at about 32 weeks to reassess and to identify risk of IUGR. After 30 weeks clinical and ultrasonographic evaluation of the cervix (> 2 cm long and closed is favourable) is carried out at intervals in some centres to guess at the likelihood of premature labour. In cases of premature labour corticosteroids and tocolytics are used (chapter 6).
4. In a case of polyhydramnios, if she is in distress, abdominal amniocentesis of 1–2 litres is done under local anesthetic, to give her relief.
5. Other complications like PIH or APH is treated (chapters 4 and 5).
6. Near term ultrasonography is useful to confirm the type of presentations and to estimate the fetal weights.

During labour: At the onset of labour, re-examine to ascertain that the presentation is vertex and the FHR is normal. Start an IV drip of 5 % dextrose saline. When the bag of membranes rupture monitor the FHR, uterine contractions and the progress of labour. If there are inadequate uterine contractions with poor progress, oxytocin infusion is given. In case of delay in delivery at the outlet, apply outlet forceps. After the first baby is born and separated, palpate the second fetus to determine the lie and presentation; if abnormal, correct it by external cephalic version (ECV) and check the FHR. The second bag of membranes is now artificially ruptured, and the second baby is delivered vaginally.

In all cases of multiple pregnancies as soon as the last baby is born, prophylactic oxytocics are given to prevent PPH. After the delivery of the placenta the mother should be observed closely for vaginal bleeding for at least an hour.

Retained second twin

If a mother is brought in after she delivers the first baby outside the hospital, examine her general condition and the abdomen.

Intact membranes

If the uterus is lax, presentation is normal and FHR is normal, rupture the second bag of membranes and infuse oxytocin. Monitor the progress and proceed with delivery as stated earlier.

If it is a breech, try ECV and if successful, perform amniotomy and infuse oxytocin. Deliver vaginally. In case ECV is not possible and the baby is of average weight, deliver by amniotomy and breech extraction (chapter 10).

If on admission, palpation confirms it is a transverse lie and the FHR is normal, ECV is followed by amniotomy. Deliver vaginally. If the ECV fails, perform amniotomy and carry out internal podalic version (IPV) and breech extraction under general anesthesia as the cervix is fully dilated.

Ruptured membranes

If the membranes of the second twin had ruptured prior to admission the mother is examined and IV fluids are administered to correct dehydration. Parenteral antibiotics are given to combat infection.

If FHR is normal, the head is not engaged, the cervix is fully or incompletely dilated, and uterine contractions are sluggish, commence oxytocin infusion. In case there is no progress in 45–60 minutes, or if fetal distress is observed, perform cesarean section.

1. Sometimes abdominal palpation shows that the second baby is presenting as a transverse lie, but has a normal FHR. If the membranes were recently ruptured and the uterus is contracting occasionally (with complete relaxation between contractions) IPV is attempted followed by breech extraction. If IPV fails, cesarean section is performed. If the second baby is large, with a malpresentation or is in distress, abdominal delivery is advised soon after admission.
2. If the fetus is dead: Head is unengaged, with inadequate uterine contractions, oxytocin infusion is commenced in anticipation of vaginal delivery. If with good uterine contractions, it is disengaged, forceps and craniotomy may be performed (chapter 11).

   If the fetus is dead and examination reveals a neglected transverse lie and hand prolapse, IV dextrose saline is given to correct dehydration. Under general anesthesia decapitation is done (chapter 11). If the physician is not experienced in embryotomy, cesarean section is done. At times an inverted T-shaped incision may be needed. Sterilisation should be done with consent if she is a parous woman. If she is a nullipara, an elective cesarean section near term is advised in her next pregnancy. After a destructive operation, the uterus must be explored to rule out any tear. In all cases of twins PPH must be prevented with an oxytocin infusion. Broad spectrum antibiotics must be given to these patients before and after the procedure.

Bibliography

Phuapradit W and Sarojpala N 2003. Multiple pregnancy. In SS Ratnam, KB Rao and S Arulkumaran (Eds). *Obstetrics and Gynecology for Postgraduates* vol 2, 2nd edn. Chennai: Orient Longman.

9. Third stage complications

The third stage of labour is the duration from the birth of the baby until complete expulsion of the placenta and membranes. It usually lasts for 5–10 minutes and rarely extends beyond 30 minutes. Complications occur unexpectedly at this stage and unless prompt action is taken, serious morbidity and sometimes mortality may occur.

Postpartum hemorrhage (PPH) accounts for about 28 per cent of maternal deaths in the developing world (approximately 125,000 per year). There are about 125 million births per year in the developing countries and so the risk of death is 1 in 1000 cases. In the developed world the risk of death is a hundred times less than in the developing countries. In the UK there were eight deaths between 1991 and 1993.

Postpartum hemorrhage may be either primary (within the first 24 hours) or secondary (after 24 hours to six weeks postpartum). Primary postpartum hemorrhage is defined as blood loss more than 500 ml in the first 24 hours. However there are problems with these definitions. Firstly, visual estimations are notoriously inaccurate. Clinical assessment underestimates blood loss by 30–50 per cent. Secondly, mothers may even be affected by blood loss that is less than 500 ml. A more practical definition will be any bleeding per vaginum following the birth of the baby till the end of puerperium, which adversely affects the general condition of the patient by causing a rise in pulse rate and lowering the blood pressure. In the western world, the focus is now on major postpartum hemorrhage (blood loss more than one litre). The incidence of PPH is approximately 5 per cent and the incidence of major PPH is about 1.3 per cent.

Physiology

The separation of the placenta is achieved by the marked reduction in the uterine surface area of the placental site following delivery, due to retraction, of the uterine muscles. By retraction, the muscle fibre length is permanently shortened. After delivery the uterus continues to contract rhythmically and the muscle fibres that stretched to accommodate the fetus are shortened by these contractions and maintained by the retractions. The relatively inelastic placenta is sheared off its attachment to the deep spongy decidual layers. Simultaneous extravasation of blood due to compression of decidual veins by uterine contractions, while the spiral arteries continue to pump blood in the intervillous space may also help in the separation of the placenta. The placenta separates either by marginal separation (Mathews–Duncan) or by central (Schultze) methods. Following placental separation, the uterine muscle fibres (arranged in a criss-cross fashion) constrict the vessels and hemostatis is achieved.

Signs of placental separation

The signs of placental separation are:

- Lengthening of the cord by 8–15 cm
- Rise of fundus and change of shape from discoid to globular form. This is due to the placenta separating and leaving the upper segment.
- Fairly brisk gush of blood due to separation.

Complications

Complications in this stage include:

1. Postpartum hemorrhage
2. Retention of placenta

3. Shock: hemorrhagic and non-hemorrhagic
4. Uterine inversion
5. Disseminated intravascular coagulation
6. Amniotic fluid embolism

POSTPARTUM HEMORRHAGE (PPH)

Postpartum hemorrhage is classified as primary and secondary. Primary hemorrhage is the hemorrhage that occurs in the first 24 hours following the birth of the baby.

Primary hemorrhage may be classified into two groups: third stage hemorrhage (bleeding before expulsion of the placenta) and bleeding after the delivery of the placenta.

Third Stage Bleeding

The principles of management are to make the uterus contract and to empty the uterus of its bleeding. Management of the retained placenta and traumatic bleeding is described in detail later in this chapter.

Causes of PPH

1. *Uterine atony:* This is the **commonest cause** (seen in 80–85 per cent of cases). It is due to failure of the normal mechanisms that ensure the hemostatic contraction and retraction of the uterine musculature. This may happen without any associated factors but is more commonly associated with:
   - Prolonged, precipitate and induced labour
   - Overdistension of the uterus with multiple pregnancy, polyhydramnios and macrosomia
   - Retained placenta, placental fragments and blood clots
   - Antepartum hemorrhage: placenta previa and abruptio placentae
   - Previous history of PPH
   - Mismanaged third stage of labour

- Structural abnormalities of the uterus, such as fibroid uterus
- Drugs: tocolytic agents and general anesthesia with halothane.
- High parity has not been shown to be a contributing factor.

2. ***Genital tract trauma:*** This is the **second commonest cause** and accounts for 10–15 per cent of cases. It could be caused by episiotomy, lacerations of perineum, vagina and cervix, laceration or rupture of the uterus, and vulvovaginal and broad ligament hematoma.
3. Acute inversion of uterus
4. Disseminated intravascular coagulation problems
5. Other causes, such as incomplete inversion of uterus or placenta accreta
6. Sheehan's syndrome

Management

Prevention: The prevention of PPH by active management of third stage of labour is discussed in other chapters. Women with high-risk factors for PPH should be identified during the antenatal period and confined in units managed by trained obstetric personnel and with easy access of blood transfusion unit. Intravenous access should be established and blood should be cross-matched during labour.

Medical management: The primary management of atonic PPH is to induce uterine contractions. One hand should be placed on the uterus abdominally and fundal massage should be started. The bladder should be catheterised and the placenta should be inspected to check its completeness. Oxytocic medications if not already given should be given. Usually oxytocin 10 units or syntometrine one vial (oxytocin 5 units and ergometrine 0.5 mg) is given IM at the delivery of the head or with the anterior shoulder. If oxytoxics have already been given, ergometrine (250 μg) should be given IV; it can be repeated after a few minutes, if necessary. In addition, an infusion of 1000 ml normal saline with 40 units of syntocinon at the rate of 100 mu/min should be started to initiate uterine contraction. These oxytocic medications usually control most of the atonic PPH. If bleeding is not controlled then 15-methyl PGF_{2a}(0.25 mg) is given intramuscularly or intramyometrially using a spinal needle. This can be repeated every 60–90 minutes several times if needed. Alternatively, another prostaglandin (misoprostol, a PGE_1 analogue) 600–1000 μg may be used. It may be given orally, vaginally or rectally. It is absorbed quickly orally; however it may cause nausea and vomiting. The vaginal route is not preferred as it will be washed away by the bleeding. However, systematic review of trials of 600 μg of oral misoprostol have shown that oxytoxin or ergometrine injections are more effective in the prevention of PPH.

Management of hypovolemia: Lost fluids should be replaced as early as possible. Rapid intravenous infusion of crystalloids (Ringer's lactate and normal saline) through two intravenous lines with 14–16 gauge cannulas should be started. In healthy non-anemic women, blood loss of upto 1500 ml can usually be managed by infusion of crystalloid. However, in anemic women or in PPH of more than 2000 ml, packed cell transfusion may be necessary. Sometimes while waiting for the blood, colloid solutions (Gelofusion) may be infused. However Gelofusion interferes with blood cross-matching and deranges blood coagulation. To prevent these complications it is prudent to start Gelofusion after blood has been sent for cross-matching. Also, only the amount necessary should be transfused. Alternatively, if fresh frozen plasma is available, it may be transfused.

Other management options

1. ***Fundal massage:*** In cases where there is a steady trickle in spite of oxytocic drugs, continuous fundal massage may help. However, this should be vigorous but not so hard as to cause trauma or pain.

2. ***Bimanual uterine compression:*** This is a painful procedure and is best used as a transient measure and in those with epidural analgesia. The vaginal hand, formed as a fist, is placed in the anterior fornix and the abdominal hand cupping and pushing down on the postero–fundal part of the uterus may provide temporary compression and reduction of bleeding.
3. ***Aortic compression:*** It may be tried in a slim patient. Here one hand pulls the uterine fundus out of the pelvis and pushes upwards and backwards across the lower part of the uterus, while the other hand directs the fundus posteriorly to compress the aorta.

The above three maneuvers are generally used as temporary measures prior to surgical management.

Surgical management: Proper assessment of each case before doing instrumental/operative delivery is essential. Only a person with appropriate competence and training should perform the operative delivery. In general, vacuum extraction is associated with less genital tract trauma than forceps. Should there be any difficulty in instrumental delivery, early recourse to cesarean section should be taken. Help from competent staff should be easily accessible.

Depending on the circumstances, the surgical management options are:

1. *Repair of lower genital tract lacerations:* Genital tract lacerations should be suspected when bleeding per vaginum persists despite the uterus being hard and well-contracted. These injuries may lead to profuse bleeding. Good light, assistance, suction and adequate exposure are necessary for high vaginal or cervical lacerations. It is usually sutured with continuous locking stitches. If difficulty is encountered in finding the apex, then a suture is placed as high as possible and then using this as traction thread the apex of the laceration is reached in stepwise fashion (Fig 9.1). At times it is best to take isolated sutures on one or the other side of the bleeding

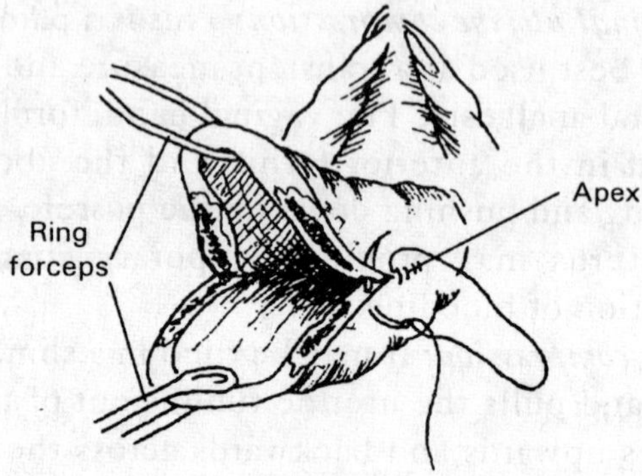

Fig 9.1 Repair of cervical tear

vaginal tear. The space between heals well with time and prevents narrowing of the upper vagina, thus allowing a better view to check if bleeding has stopped.

2. *Cervical lacerations* can be identified by using sponge forceps. The anterior lip is grasped at the 12 o'clock region and the second forceps is placed at 2–3 o'clock position. The tissues in between are inspected and then the first forceps is moved to the 5–6 o'clock region; the whole region of the cervical lips is inspected in this way. Lacerations without bleeding need not be sutured. Bleeding lacerations are sutured by interrupted stitches. Sometimes leaving the area clamped with sponge forceps for some time controls the oozing/bleeding.
3. *Paragenital hematoma:* They are classified as infralevator and supralevator. The infralevator group involves vulval, perineal, paravaginal abdominal hematomas occurring in the ischiorectal fossa. The supralevator hematoma bulges into the walls of upper vagina and spreads upwards and laterally in the broad ligaments.
   a. Vulval and paravaginal hematomas present with pain, swelling and features of hypovolemia. These hematomas should be incised and clots evacuated. Active bleeding points should be located and ligated. In most cases, no active bleeding points are

found but oozing areas are oversewn. The area is repaired in layers and the vagina is packed with gauze and a Foley's catheter is inserted in the bladder.

b. Supralevator hematomas are rare but occur if a blood vessel ruptures above the pelvic fascia and bleeds between the leaves of the broad ligament. It presents with pain, tachycardia and progressive anemia; on palpation the uterus is found pushed to one side by the broad ligament mass. Rupture of the uterus should always be excluded. Treatment involves management of hypovolemia with intravenous crystalloid, colloid solution and blood. If uterine rupture has been excluded and the patient is stable, conservative management with close observation may be continued. However, if there is continued deterioration then either angiographic embolisation of the branches of the involved internal iliac artery or laparotomy with evacuation of the hematoma and ligature of active bleeding points have to be tried first. However, in some cases hysterectomy has to be performed. If uterine trauma is present, efforts should be made to repair it before performing a hysterectomy.

4. *Uterine tamponade:* After years of disrepute, uterine packing has recently found favour again in specific cases. This requires general anesthesia and very tight and systematic packing of the uterine cavity with a gauze roll. The vagina is packed and a Foley's catheter is placed. Recently, packing has been tried after placing a plastic drape, shaped like a bag, which helps easy removal of the pack. Other methods involve use of Sengstaken–Blakemore tube and the use of balloon. The balloon portions are inflated and kept in place for 12–24 hours. Continuous infusion of oxytocin is started and antibiotics are prescribed.

5. *Major vessel embolisation:* If facilities are available,

angiographic embolisation of the branches of the internal iliac artery is used to successfully control hemorrhage from uterine atony and trauma to cervix, paracolpos and upper vagina. It may be done under local anesthesia under sedation. The bleeding vessels are identified by extravasation of the contrast agent and blocked by injection of gelfoam particles. A catheter is guided, through the femoral artery under angiographic control, to the aortic bifurcation and then in turn to each of the internal iliac vessels and its branches.

6. *Major vessel ligation:* The first step in this procedure is to do a combination of uterine and ovarian artery ligation. The advantage of this procedure is that it can be done by general obstetricians. The bladder is pushed deep down and using a large curved needle and No. 1 absorbable suture the needle is passed through the myometrium from the front to the back, and then through the avascular portion of the broad ligament to encircle the ascending branch of the uterine artery. An encircling suture is also passed in the manner stated just below the uterine attachment of the utero-ovarian ligament. The sutures are repeated on either side. This surgery can be performed safely and swiftly.

   Internal iliac ligation may also be tried. However, this is a more complicated procedure and is more suitable for hemorrhage from injury to cervix, paracolpos and upper vagina, uterine atony and placenta accreta. Before initiating it, the patient should be examined under anesthesia and direct sutures to bleeding areas vaginally should be attempted. The descending branch of the uterine arteries supplies the cervix, vagina and paracolpos. The retroperitoneal space is entered in between the round ligament and the fallopian tube, and the point of bifurcation of the common iliac artery is identified. The ureter and its attached peritoneum are identified and reflected laterally. The external iliac artery is identified first; then the internal iliac artery is lifted with Babcock clamps and tied with non-absorbable sutures (passing it from the lateral to the medial side). Great care must be taken not to injure the underlying veins. This procedure reduces the pulse pressure by about 85 per cent, making it approximately similar to that of the venous system. It is effective in about 40–50 per cent of persons in whom medical management and uterine artery ligation have failed. This procedure also restricts the access for future angiographic embolisation of vessels.

7. *Uterine compression sutures:* Recently, various types of compression sutures have been used to control the bleeding and to conserve the uterus. The first of these was described by Lynch; it requires opening of the lower uterine segment. Others have used compression sutures without having to make a uterine incision.
8. *Hysterectomy:* If all of the above measures fail, hysterectomy should be performed. It is always better to make the decision of hysterectomy earlier than at a very late stage as the patient's condition deteriorates abruptly.
9. *Retained placenta:* The incidence of the retained placenta thirty minutes after delivery is 2–4 per cent. Active management reduces the placental delivery time by half compared to the time taken after conservative management. The longer the placenta is retained, the greater is the risk of postpartum hemorrhage. In the absence of active bleeding, the timing depends on the availability of safe anesthesia, which should be arranged within 30–60 minutes. It has also been noted that in half of the cases, the placenta deliver spontaneously in that time. However, in the presence of bleeding, arrangements for manual removal under anesthesia (Fig 9.2) should be made as soon as possible.

The causes of retained placenta: Uterine atony or constriction rings may cause retention of the placenta even though it has separated from the uterine wall. Retained adherent placenta is due to failure of the

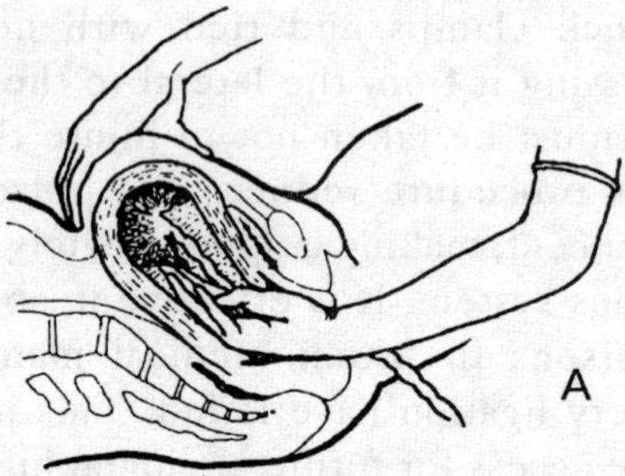

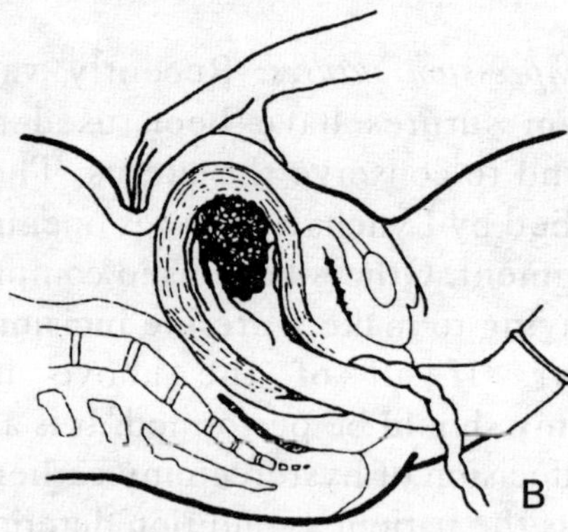

Fig 9.2 A. Supporting the fundus while detaching the placenta
B. Withdrawing the hand from the uterus

separation through the decidua spongiosa layer or due to pathological adherence resulting from deficient decidual reaction allowing invasion of the myometrium by the trophoblast. This is more likely if the uterine site has previously been affected by surgery, trauma or infection. The degrees of pathological adherence are placental accreta (adherence to myometrium), placenta increta (invading the myometrium) and placenta percreta (penetrating through the myometrium to the serosal layer). Due to poor decidual reaction placental adherence is more commonly noted in cases of placenta previa.

Management of retained placenta is by manual removal

under anesthesia. If the patient is bleeding, an intravenous oxytocin drip is started and the placenta is removed as follows:

- Under suitable anesthesia the right hand is placed in the vagina and the cord followed up to the cervix. The left hand firmly fixes the uterine fundus.
- The fingers and thumb of the uterine hand are kept extended and used as one unit to find the lower margin of the placenta and the plane of cleavage. The placenta is gradually separated with a sideways movement of the fingers until the whole placenta is separated. Once the placenta has been completely removed, it is grasped and slowly removed through the cervix and then the uterus is re-explored to make sure that there are no remnants of the placenta. The cervix and vagina are checked and any lacerations sutured. Antibiotics are given to prevent intrauterine infections and an oxytocin drip is started to maintain uterine contraction and retraction.
- In case of pathological adherence the placenta is removed piecemeal from those sites and effective uterine contractions are achieved with oxytocics. In cases where the placenta is totally morbidly adherent, hysterectomy is indicated in parous women and in patients desirous of bearing more children, the umbilical cord is cut as high as possible. The placenta is left to autolyse under antibiotic cover. In such situations oral methotrexate has also been used to dissolve the placenta.
- If sufficient uterine relaxation is not obtained by regional anesthesia, intravenous nitroglycerine may be used.
- In some case of retained placenta an IU injection of 10–20 units of oxytocin mixed with 20 ml of normal saline has been used to deliver the placenta. The

results of this technique are mixed and inconclusive but since there are no side effects it may be worth trying this before resorting to anesthesia.

10. *Acute uterine inversion:* This is a rare condition; the incidence varies between 1 in 2000 to 1 in 50,000 deliveries. Inversion may be incomplete (the fundus is inverted but does not protrude through the cervix) or complete (the inverted fundus passes through the vagina and lies in the vagina or outside the introitus).

    Mismanagement of the third stage is the commonest cause of uterine inversion. However, very rarely, it may occur spontaneously with sudden rise of intra-abdominal pressure from coughing and vomiting even in a relaxed uterus. It may also follow rapid removal of placenta during manual removal.

    The diagnosis is usually obvious with the sudden appearance of a boggy mass in the vagina or at the introitus. This is associated with sudden onset of lower abdominal pain, profound hypotension, bradycardia and pallor. There is neurogenic shock (due to the traction on the infundibulo-pelvic ligament) but it is followed by hypovolemic shock from the associated bleeding. Incomplete inversion may be difficult to diagnose but it is usually associated with continued bleeding. A submucous fibroid protruding through the cervix should be excluded.

    If the condition is to be prevented, Crede's method of delivery of the placenta should not be used. While delivering the placenta, there should be no cord traction in a relaxed uterus and countertraction should be provided during delivery of the placenta in a contracted uterus.

    Management of acute inversion includes pain relief with morphine/pethidine to counteract neurogenic shock, setting up of two intravenous lines with transfusion of crystalloids for hypovolemia. Four units of blood should be cross-matched. Efforts should be made to replace the uterus immediately; during that process the part that inverted last should be replaced first (Fig 9.3). If successful, a bolus of an oxytocic should be given to initiate uterine contraction. If unsuccessful, the patient has to be transferred to the theatre and under general anesthesia (halothane), the uterus is manually replaced. The placenta is removed only after correction of inversion. Remove your hand only after the uterus has contracted fully. Oxytocin infusion should be given for 8–12 hours and the uterus should be explored for intactness. Sometimes tocolytic agents may be helpful in correction of inversion and IV nitroglycerine may be given in the dose of 100–200 mg every 2–3 minutes until there is good relaxation.

The hydrostatic method of O'Sullivan may be necessary if the above methods fail. The principle of this method is distension of the vaginal fornices with fluid. This pulls (outwards) on the constricting cervical ring and thus allows replacement of the inversion. Having excluded tears in the vagina, cervix and uterus, a douche nozzle is placed in the posterior fornix, while the other hand seals the vaginal orifice. Upto five litres of saline (warmed to body temperature) may be needed. In

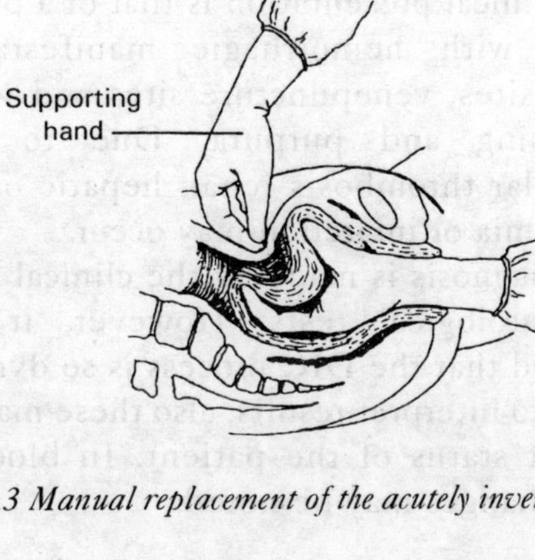

Fig 9.3 Manual replacement of the acutely inverted uterus

chronic cases of incomplete inversion, laparotomy is required and traction is provided to the inverted fundus with tenacula (Huntington's technique). If this is not successful, the constriction ring is incised posteriorly to allow correction of inversion and then the incised portion is sutured.

11. *Disseminated intravascular coagulation:* In health, there is a balance between the coagulation and fibrinolytic system, which ensures hemostasis. However, in disseminated intravascular coagulation (DIC) there is excess and generalised coagulation due to release of thromboplastins into the maternal circulation. This causes excessive consumption and eventual depletion of coagulation factors. The fibrinolytic system is also activated and the breakdown of fibrin forms fibrin degradation products (FDP). These inhibit both thrombin and platelet function, thus aggravating the coagulation problem. DIC in pregnancy is always secondary to another initiating factor. Conditions that may cause DIC include massive blood loss leading to hypovolemic shock in abruptio placentae, massive PPH and uterine rupture. It has also been noted in amniotic fluid embolism and severe preeclampsia, eclampsia, septic abortion, retained dead fetus, hydatidiform mole and in massive blood transfusion.

    The clinical presentation is that of a primary cause associated with hemorrhagic manifestations from operatives sites, venepuncture sites and with signs of easy bruising and purpura. Due to widespread microvascular thrombosis renal, hepatic or pulmonary organ ischemia or infarction may occur.

    The diagnosis is made by the clinical features and after hematological tests. However, it should be remembered that the DIC process is so dynamic that it is difficult to interpret results; also these may not reflect the current status of the patient. In blood tests the following changes may be noted:

a. Progressive fall of platelets
b. Both prothrombin time and thrombin time are usually prolonged.
c. Fibrinogen degradation products (FDP) levels rise and levels above 80 mg/dl are very suggestive of the diagnosis. This may remain elevated for 24–48 hours even after the DIC has been controlled.
d. Red blood cells become abnormally shaped and fragmented as they pass through the fibrin mesh and a blood smear may show these abnormally shaped schizocytes.
e. Microangiopathic hemolytic anemia may develop due to widespread destruction of the red blood cells and this may result in hemolysis and hemoglobinuria.
f. Fibrinogen levels may fall to a non-pregnant range. In severe DIC, the level falls below 150 mg/dl.

The management of DIC should be multidisciplinary, involving the obstetrician, hematologist, anesthetist and the midwife. DIC may develop and progress very rapidly. The mainstay of treatment is to treat the initiating cause. Once this is controlled, the patient's circulation should be restored and maintained along with the replacement of procoagulants. The principles of maintaining circulation and organ perfusion include:

- Rapid infusion of crystalloid, colloid and packed red cells.
- Oxygen by face mask, endotracheal intubation and ventilation may be required.
- Circulation should be monitored by central venous pressure line. If this is not possible hematocrit levels should be kept above 30 and urinary output above 30 ml/hour.
- Replacement of procoagulants should be guided by hematologists.
- Fresh frozen plasma (FFP) contains all the clotting

factors and usually one unit of FFP is given after initial transfusion of five units of blood. Thereafter one unit of FFP is given for every two units of packed cell transfusion

- Cryoprecipitate is rich in fibrinogen, von Willebrand factor and factors VIII and XIII. It is given in case of severe hypofibrinogenemia.
- Platelet transfusion may be necessary in cases of severe thrombocytopenia and each unit may increase the count by 5000–10,000.
- Under the guidance of a hematologist, antithrombin III may be given provided the initiating cause has been managed and the circulation and organ perfusion maintained; these patients recover completely.

Other causes of collapse

Other causes of collapse within 24 hours of delivery includes pulmonary embolism, amniotic fluid embolism, anesthetic complications, cardiac failure in patients with pre-existing cardiac conditions (cardiomyopathy, valvular diseases or ischemic diseases), eclampsia, cerebrovascular accidents, hypoglycemia, septicemia and pneumothorax. All these conditions require specific and multidisciplinary management and are described in other chapters.

SECONDARY POSTPARTUM HEMORRHAGE

Secondary postpartum hemorrhage is defined as sudden loss of fresh blood from the genital tract after the first 24 hours and within six weeks of delivery. The common causes are retained remnants of cotyledon and membrane, separation of the slough over genital (uterine, cervical or vaginal) laceration and subinvolution of the placental site due to infection. Secondary hemorrhage following cesarean section usually occurs between 10 and 14 days and is usually due to separation of the slough exposing a bleeding vessel, or from granulation tissue. Withdrawal or breakthrough bleeding while taking hormonal contraceptives may also contribute to secondary PPH. The other rare causes include choriocarcinoma, placental polyp, infected fibroid polyp or cervical cancer.

The patient presents with bright red and varying amount of blood loss with features of sepsis and anemia. After general and abdominal examination, an internal examination should be conducted and genital swabs should be taken. Uterine involution and status of the cervical os should be noted.

The principles of management are to assess the amount of blood loss and replace it, and to identify the cause of PPH and manage it appropriately. An ultrasound scan should be performed to rule out retained products and antibiotics given to protect from aerobic and anerobic organisms (chapter 18). If retained products are detected, they should be evacuated under anesthesia and great care should be taken during the procedure as chances of perforation in puerperal uterus are high. All tissues obtained should be sent for histology. If no products are detected in the scan and the cervical os is closed, the patient is conservatively managed with antibiotics.

Bleeding from cervicovaginal lacerations is controlled by hemostatic sutures under antibiotic cover. Care should be taken during the procedure as the tissues are friable. Secondary hemorrhage following cesarean section can, at times, be severe and cause shock. Most patients present with warning bleeding, which should not be ignored. If conservative treatment is not successful laparotomy has to be performed. This may result in exploration of the cesarean wound or ligation of the internal iliac arteries. Some women may need hysterectomy, and will therefore require large amounts of blood transfusion.

Conclusion

Third stage complications can be life threatening and events progress very rapidly. Help should be sought early and each case should be managed efficiently to prevent an adverse outcome. Fire drills regarding the management of third stage complications should be undertaken in obstetric units from time to time.

Bibliography

Department of Health, Welsh Office 1996. Report of confidential enquiries into maternal deaths in the United Kingdom 1991–1993. London: HMSO.

Raghavan KS 1995. Postpartum hemorrhage. In: U Krishna, B Coyaji et al (Eds) *Safe Motherhood*. Mumbai: FOGSI, 201–210.

McDonald S, Prendiville WJ and Elbourne D 1999. Prophylactic syntometrine versus oxytocin for delivery of the placenta (Cochrane Review). In: *The Cochrane Library*, Issue 2. Oxford: Update Software.

Gulmezoglu AM 1999. Prostaglandins for prevention of postpartum hemorrhage (Cochrane Review). In: *The Cochrane Library*, Issue 2. Oxford Update Software.

Bamigboye AA, Hofmeyr GJ and Merrell DA 1998. Rectal misoprostol in the prevention of postpartum hemorrhage: a placebo controlled trial. *Am J Obstet Gynecol* 179: 1043–1046.

Lynch C, Coker A, Lawal AH, Abu J et al 1997. The B–Lynch surgical technique for the control of massive postpartum hemorrhage: an alternative to hysterectomy? Five cases reported. *Br J Obstet Gynaecol* 104: 372–375.

Villar J, Gulmezoghi A et al 2002. Review of R & T of misoprostol in prevention of PPH. *Obstet Gynecol* 100: 1301–12.

10. Vaginal operative deliveries

When a spontaneous vaginal delivery is not possible, the parturient may require the assistance of a health attendant to complete the delivery either abdominally, by cesarean section or by vaginal operative procedures (depending on several factors).

Incidence

Until a decade ago, more vaginal operative deliveries were performed compared to cesarean sections. With liberalisation of cesarean sections, the number of vaginal operative deliveries is declining. In a large multicentric study of over 22,000 deliveries, 14 per cent had a cesarean section and 4 per cent had vaginal operative deliveries (3.5 per cent forceps/ vacuum and 0.5 per cent vaginal breech).

Types of vaginal operative deliveries

1. Forceps or vacuum extractions
2. Vaginal delivery in cases of shoulder dystocia or arrested shoulders
3. Vaginal breech delivery
4. Internal podalic version in transverse lie or shoulder presentation
5. Trachelotomy
6. Destructive operations like craniotomy, decapitation and craniocentesis.

FORCEPS DELIVERY

The obstetric forceps has been in use for almost 400 years. The original instrument has been improved by i) changing the solid blade to a fenestrated type making it lighter and less traumatic; ii) addition of pelvic curve to the original cephalic curve; this helps traction along the pelvic axis; iii) introduction of longer handles and more secure locks.

It is a useful instrument to achieve completion of delivery by traction applied to cephalic presentations (usually vertex, or face in mentoanterior), and in rare cases, to the head emerging later in breech delivery.

Fetal indications

1. Fetal distress as indicated by changes in FHR or meconium stained liquor
2. Delayed second stage.

Maternal indications

1. Maternal conditions like PIH, or heart disease, to cut short the second stage.
2. When the mother is exhausted or the contractions are less forceful.
3. Delayed second stage due to rigid perineum or in those under epidural anesthesia.

The conditions to be satisfied before forceps application are: cervix must be fully dilated, membranes ruptured, vertex presentation, head 1/5th or less felt per abdomen, uterine contractions should be present, local or pudendal block anesthesia is needed. Descent of the fetal head with contractions and bearing down apart indicates the possibility of vaginal delivery. An attempt should be made to palpate the fetal ear; this will indicate whether the head is deliverable and will also indicate the position of the vertex.

Procedure of forceps delivery

Assemble the forceps first and check that it locks well. After lubricating the blades, the left blade is held in the left hand and carefully inserted along the left vaginal wall between the head and the fingers of the right hand (inserted beside the head earlier). The right blade is then held in the right hand and inserted similarly on the right side between the head and the left hand. The handles are depressed and the blades locked. The saggital suture should be midway between the blades to indicate correct application. Then steady traction is applied downwards and backwards with uterine contractions and bearing down efforts till the head begins to emerge; the forceps is then removed and the delivery accomplished (Fig 10.1).

Types of forceps delivery

1. Outlet forceps: This is the most common type of forceps delivery. The forceps is applied to the fully rotated fetal head when it has reached the perineum and is seen at vaginal introitus between contractions.
2. Low forceps: Here, the leading edge of fetal head is at +2 or just above it (with rotation occasionally incomplete as in transverse position)
3. Mid-forceps: This is rare. Here, the leading edge of the fetal head is above the +2 station. It is often malrotated and needs a skilled and experienced obstetrician. In view of the station and malrotation it may be traumatic. Delivery by cesarean section is preferable to a difficult mid-forceps.
4. High forceps: This is never used since the head is not engaged, except as a preliminary to a craniotomy in a dead fetus by a person experienced in this technique.
5. Trial of forceps is performed in the operation theatre. With traction if no descent is noticed the attempt is abandoned and cesarean section is done immediately.
6. Failed forceps: The causes are genuine CPD, malposition or very early application of forceps before the head is low enough (in rare cases) or if the cervix is not fully dilated.

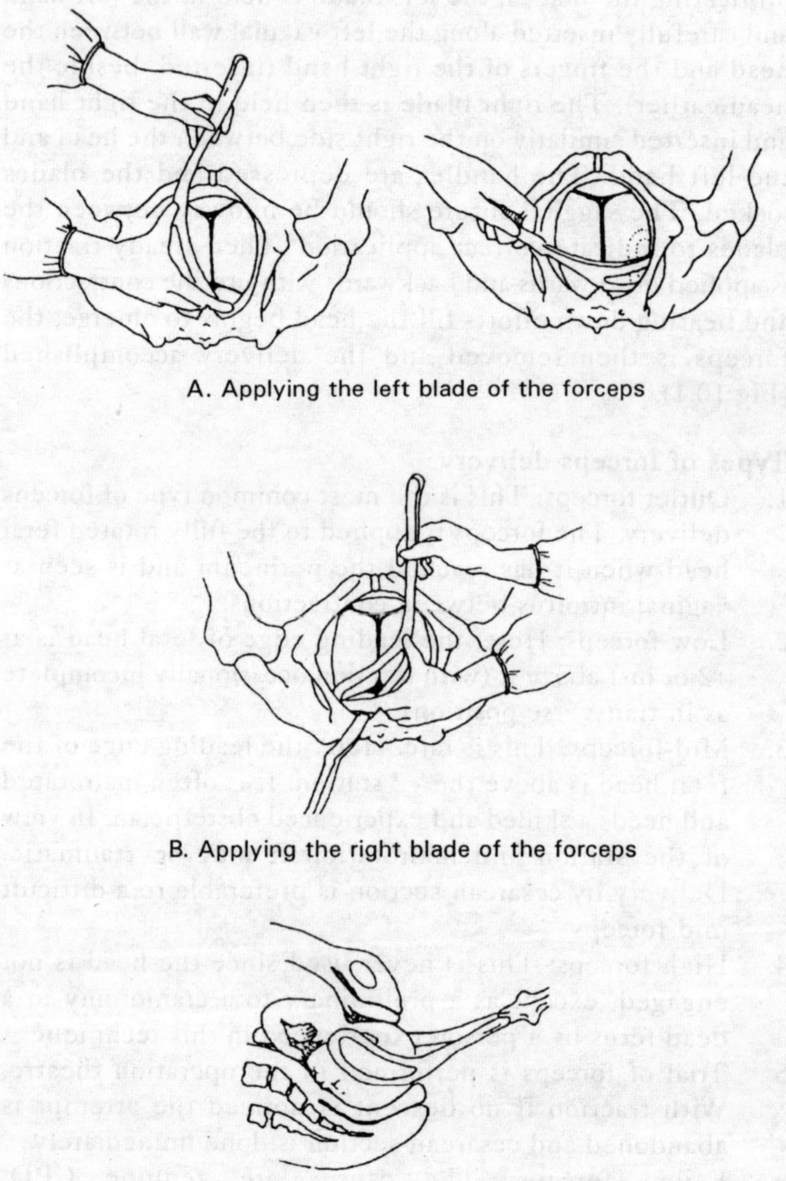

A. Applying the left blade of the forceps

B. Applying the right blade of the forceps

C. Locking and applying traction

Fig 10.1 Forceps delivery

Complications

Fetal complications

1. Injury to face, scalp and/or cephalhematoma
2. Facial palsy due to pressure on the nerve as it comes out of the stylomastoid foramen
3. Intracranial hemorrhage with its sequelae
4. Rarely, depressed fracture skull.

Maternal complications

1. Vaginal lacerations due to forceps rotation; cervical tear with traumatic PPH
2. Injury to the urethra
3. Rarely, rupture of the uterus.

VACUUM EXTRACTOR

This is a safer alternative to forceps delivery. For outlet delivery with a vacuum extractor, no anesthetic is needed as it does not distend or lacerate the vagina. It consists of a cup (metal or preferably silicone) connected through a tube and a handle to a manually or electrically operated vacuum pump. The cup is attached with its knob towards the occiput (flexion point) to help in the direction of traction. The 'flexion point' is in the midline along the sagittal suture just in front of the occiput. The cup should be applied in the midline with the posterior margin of the cup 1–2 cm anterior to the occiput (Fig 10.2). The occipito-transverse and posterior positions thus warrant a 'posterior cup' for easy maneuverability. A negative pressure of 0.8 kg/cm^2 is created and traction applied at right angles to the cup intermittently with uterine contractions and bearing down efforts. The duration of traction should not exceed 15 minutes to avoid injury to the fetal scalp or maternal soft parts. As soon as the head emerges, vacuum is released and the cup is detached. The 'chignon' or caput disappears in 24–48 hours.

The indications and conditions that should be satisfied

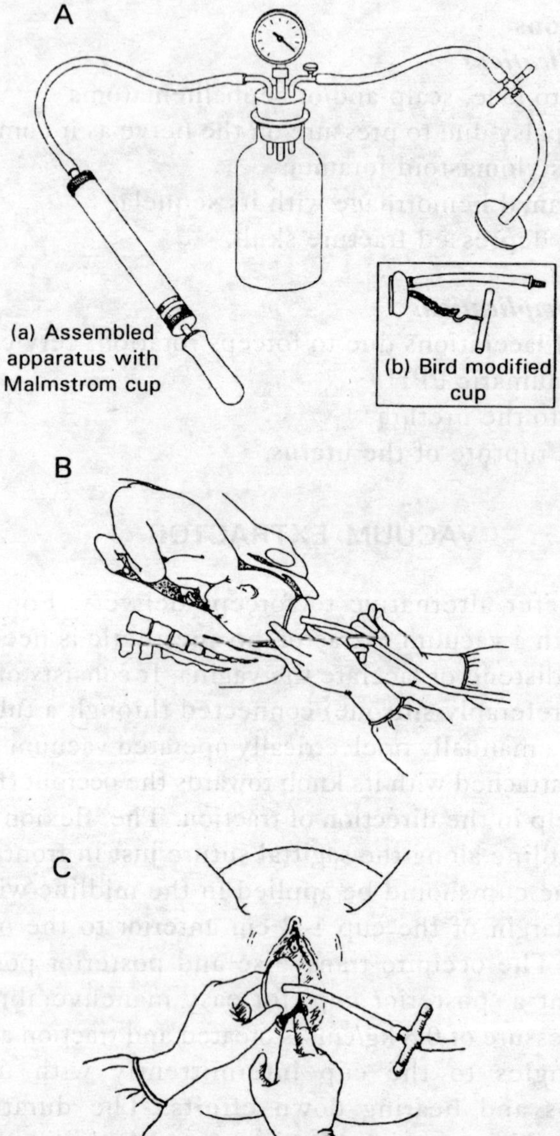

Fig 10.2 A. Vacuum extractor
B. Applying Malmstrom cup C. Applying traction

for using a vacuum extractor are the same as for forceps delivery. It can be used only for vertex presentation, mainly for traction but also for autorotation. An experienced obstetrician could use it in rare cases when the cervix is not fully dilated in a multiparous woman.

Complications

Cephalhematoma is more common with a vacuum extractor (5 per cent) than with a forceps. Rarely, retinal hemorrhages may occur. Maternal morbidity is negligible. Failed vacuum extractions may be due to

- Defective pump and leakage of air
- High station of the head
- Midcavity dystocia
- Improper application (of cup or position).

SHOULDER DYSTOCIA

This is described as difficulty in delivering the shoulders after the birth of the fetal head. It is a very serious emergency as the delivery may result in fetal hypoxia, brachial nerve injury (C5 to T1) or fetal death.

Incidence

It is seen in about 0.5 per cent of all deliveries.

Etiology

In normal labour, the shoulders enter the pelvis, either transversely or obliquely, passing behind the pubis, and rotate internally at the level of the mid-pelvis prior to their delivery. In shoulder dystocia, the shoulders try to enter the pelvis in the anteroposterior diameter, fail to rotate and get arrested at the brim. Usually, the anterior shoulder is impacted over the symphysis pubis. Rarely, there could be bilateral shoulder impaction with the posterior shoulder impacted over the sacral promontory. It is usually seen in macrosomic infants (fetal weight over 4000 g) and in diabetic mothers.

In a typical case the baby's head is just delivered, the cheeks and chin are born, followed by the chin being pulled back against the perineum ('turtle neck syndrome') and the face fails to rotate externally. Attempt to deliver the shoulders with moderate downward traction on the head is usually unsuccessful. Severe traction may cause brachial plexus injury especially with excessive downward traction (Fig 10.3). The baby tries to breathe and becomes cyanotic.

Complications

Due to delay in the delivery, anoxia may lead to hypoxic-

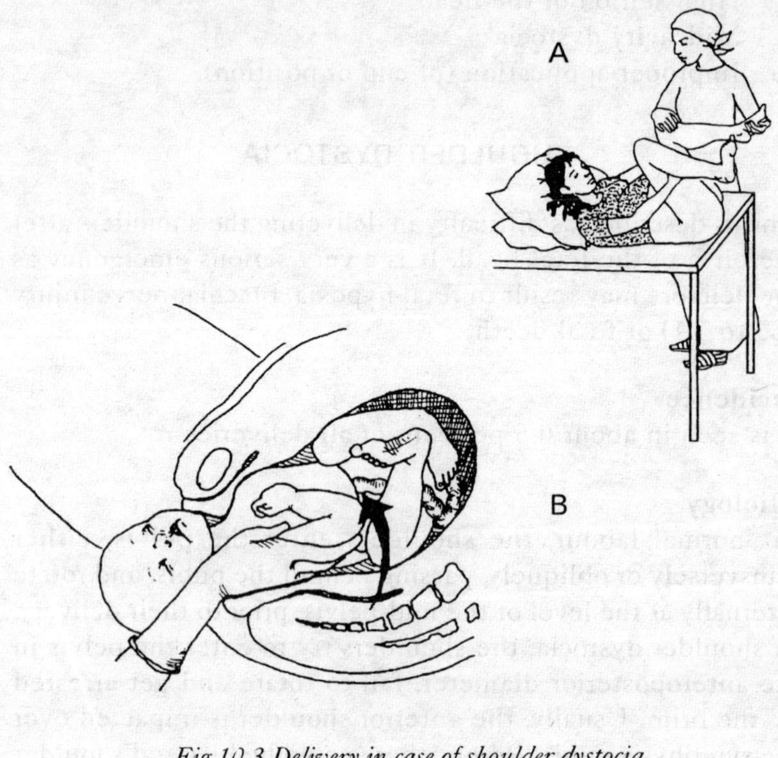

Fig 10.3 Delivery in case of shoulder dystocia
A. Assistant pushing flexed knees firmly towards chest.
B. Grasping the humerus of the arm that is posterior and sweeping the arm across the chest

ischemic encephalopathy, and forcible attempts at delivery may cause brachial nerve palsy (C5 to T1) or fracture of the humerus. Undue delay results in neurological damage or stillbirth and possibly to medicolegal problems.

Management

Prevention: It is advisable to perform an elective cesarean in all mothers with previous history of shoulder dystocia, especially in the presence of macrosomia and diabetes. Ultrasonography may help in assessing the fetal weight as well as the transthoracic diameter. If this diameter exceeds the biparietal diameter by 1.6 cm, a cesarean section should be performed. It should also be preferred in all cases where the baby is large and vaginal delivery involves delay in the late first stage and delayed descent of the fetal head into the pelvis. In the second stage of labour, a cesarean section should be considered, especially if instrumental vaginal delivery is contemplated.

When the arrest of the shoulders is anticipated or when faced with such an emergency, an experienced obstetrician, anesthetist, additional assistants and a pediatrician should be readily available.

1. First enlarge the episiotomy to create more space for any intravaginal manipulations.
2. Place the woman in McRobert's position: both thighs are abducted, rotated outwards, and flexed with the thighs touching the sides of the abdomen thus helping the posterior shoulder to move backwards and for the anterior shoulder to enter the pelvis. If this does not help, directed suprapubic pressure is applied (by an assistant) with the palm of the hand posteriorly and laterally in the direction the baby is facing, in order to adduct the shoulders and to rotate them into the oblique diameter of the pelvis. At the same time, gentle traction and rotation is applied to the head and neck below, to assist the anterior shoulder to enter the pelvis. In 90 per cent of the cases, this is adequate.

3. If this has not been helpful, the hand is inserted posteriorly and pressure is applied to the anterior aspect of the posterior shoulder in the direction of the fetal back (Wood's procedure) along with external rotation to get the shoulders to the oblique diameter of the pelvis.
4. If this too fails, introduce the hand into the hollow of the sacrum and deliver the posterior shoulder. The upper arm is pushed forwards and the arm flexed at the elbow; the forearm is brought down followed by upper arm. At times this may lead to fracture of the humerus, but it could be treated easily.

In case of an anencephalic or dead fetus, cleidotomy or fracture of clavicle is the procedure of choice.

BREECH DELIVERY

In chapter 7, the role of cesarean section and vaginal delivery of uncomplicated breech presentations has been discussed. In breech presentations, the assisted breech delivery is more common than breech extraction.

In assisted breech delivery, the baby is allowed to be born spontaneously till the umbilicus. The emergence of the shoulders and the head are assisted by the physician. In the first stage, the mother is watched and when the membranes rupture, a vaginal examination is done to determine the cervical dilatation, station of the breech and to rule out cord prolapse. In the second stage she is encouraged to bear down only when the breech is low in the 'perineal phase'. As the breech distends the perineum and does not recede between contractions, an episiotomy is done to assist the breech delivery (Fig 10.4). In complete breech the legs may be hooked out as they appear. In frank breech their release is assisted when the knees appear by slight abduction of the thighs followed by outward pressure under the knee to flex it and deliver the legs. With subsequent contractions, the buttocks, lower back and the shoulder blades are seen. With

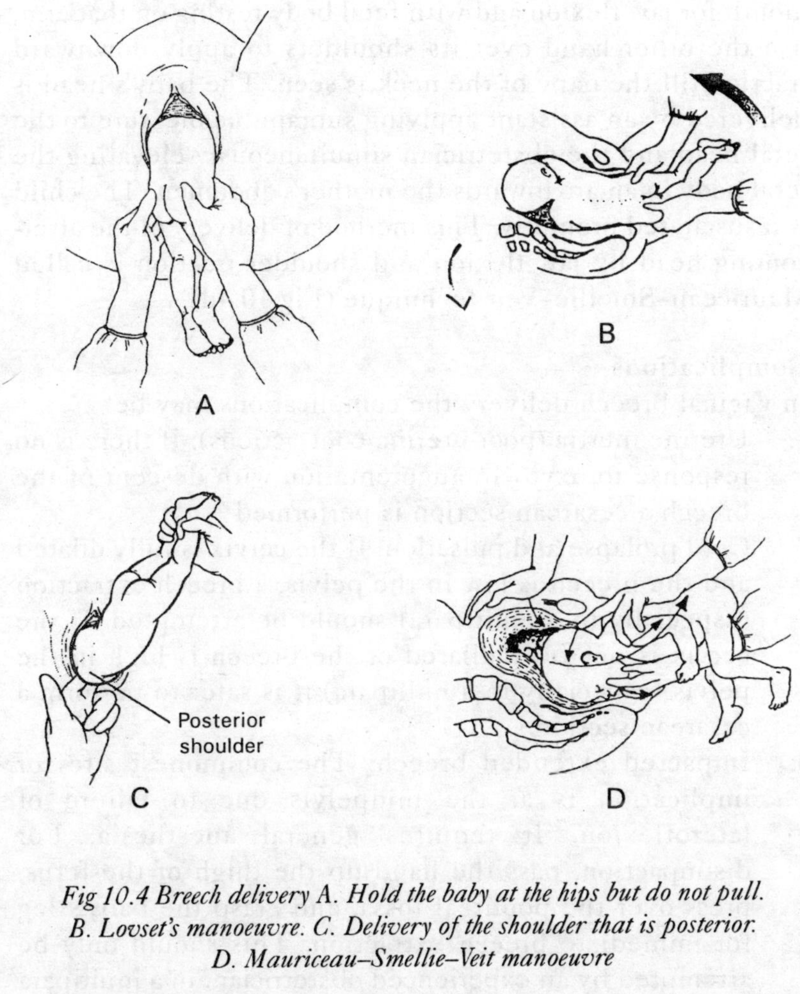

Fig 10.4 Breech delivery A. Hold the baby at the hips but do not pull. B. Lovset's manoeuvre. C. Delivery of the shoulder that is posterior. D. Mauriceau–Smellie–Veit manoeuvre

a steady traction over the hips, slight rotation of the body and the mother bearing down, the anterior shoulder and arm are seen at the vulva and are released. Rotation of the baby in the opposite direction helps to relieve the other arm.

After the shoulders are delivered the back of the body should be made to face upwards. The head enters the pelvis due to the weight of its trunk. With the index and ring fingers over the maxilla and midfinger (of the left hand) in the baby's mouth for jaw flexion and with fetal body resting on that arm, use the other hand over its shoulders to apply downward traction till the nape of the neck is seen. The baby's head is delivered by an assistant applying suprapubic pressure to the fetal head and the obstetrician simultaneously elevating the fetal body in an arc towards the mother's abdomen. The child is resuscitated promptly. This method of delivery of the after-coming head by jaw flexion and shoulder traction is called Mauriceau–Smellie–Veit technique (Fig 10.4d).

Complications

In vaginal breech delivery the complications may be:

1. Uterine inertia (poor uterine contractions): If there is no response to oxytocin augmentation with descent of the breech a cesarean section is performed
2. Cord prolapse and pulsation: If the cervix is fully dilated and the breech is low in the pelvis, a breech extraction (especially in a multipara) should be attempted. If the cervix is not fully dilated or the breech is high in the pelvis (especially in a nullipara) it is safer to perform a cesarean section.
3. Impacted extended breech: The commonest site for implication is at the midpelvis due to failure of lateroflexion. It requires general anesthesia. For disimpaction, pass the hand up the thigh of the fetus, press over the popliteal fossa, and grasp the baby's leg for immediate breech extraction. This should only be attempted by an experienced obstetrician, in a multipara who is presenting with a small or average size baby. A cesarean section is preferred if there is no spontaneous descent. If the impaction is at the brim, the cause may be fetopelvic disproportion; this requires a cesarean section. Impaction at the outlet is tackled by finger traction at the groin, only when the breech is distending the perineum.
4. Difficulty in delivery of the shoulders is overcome by the Lovset procedure. It is based on the principle that when

the anterior shoulder is behind the symphysis pubis, the posterior shoulder is below the sacral promontory. Hence, when the trunk is rotated through 180 degrees, the posterior shoulder is beneath the symphysis pubis when the arm is hooked out. The other shoulder is now rotated in the opposite direction and finally the head is delivered as described earlier.

5. Difficulty in delivering the after-coming head: The causes are incomplete dilatation of the cervix, contracted pelvis, deflexed head and hydrocephalus. If none of these factors are present, it could be delivered by forceps. If the baby is dead it requires craniotomy; if hydrocephalic decompression is required craniocentesis should be attempted.

Breech extraction

This should only be attempted by an obstetrician experienced in the technique. It may be suitable for multiparas, and where the breech is low in the pelvis and the size of the fetus is small or of average size. When the cervix is fully dilated, and there is an indication for immediate delivery of the breech (as in cord prolapse, fetal distress etc.) under general anesthesia after a preliminary episiotomy, the foot is grasped from the vagina and traction applied to it. The breech is then delivered with back to the front. On further traction care is taken to avoid deflexion of the head. The rest of the baby is delivered as described earlier (pp 120).

Internal podalic version

Internal podalic version is an intrauterine manipulation for turning the fetus by bringing down the podalic pole or the feet. An unfavourable presentation (for example, shoulder) is converted to a more favorable one like breech by this procedure. Since it caries a risk of uterine rupture the patient has to be assessed and the delivery conducted by an experienced obstetrician in the setting of an operating theatre with an anesthetist present (should a cesarean section become necessary).

Incidence

Incidence is less than 0.5 per cent.

Indications

In modern obstetrics, internal podalic version is restricted to selected cases of transverse lie (rarely) and the second of twins (chapters 7 and 8).

The conditions to be satisfied for internal podalic version are that the patient should be in labour, the cervix should be fully dilated, the membranes recently ruptured, the uterus contracting and relaxed in intervals. (In a case of previous cesarean section internal podalic version is contraindicated.)

Procedure

Ideally internal podalic version is done in the second of twins presenting as a transverse lie when external cephalic version fails or when membranes rupture with prolapse of a hand or cord. The fetus is mapped out by palpation under general anesthesia and the surgeon introduces his hand into the uterus, identifies the foot by the heel, grasps it and pulls it down. As the cervix is fully dilated, breech extraction is done carefully; the child is resuscitated by an experienced pediatrician.

If the cervix is incompletely dilated, and there is cord prolapse with absent pulsation when the membranes rupture in a transverse lie, only IPV is done and the breech is delivered later to avoid traumatic PPH.

Complications

Rupture of the uterus may take place if the internal podalic version is done late in labour, on a grand multipara, done forcefully or when good contractions are present.

Trachelotomy

Very rarely, in a parous woman the fetal vertex might descend below the level of the ischial spines. However, an edematous prolapsed cervix may be just over 7 cm and does not dilate further. In such cases, if there is no contraction of the cervix at the lower levels, the cervix may be cut between clamps at 2, 6, and 10 o'clock positions. Later, only if necessary, the forceps is applied and the baby delivered. After the birth of the placenta, the clamps are replaced by sutures. This procedure is rarely warranted and should be done in the operating theatre with considerable care. There is always the possibility of the incision extending upwards and causing uterine rupture, pelvic hemorrhage and hematoma.

DESTRUCTIVE OPERATIONS

Destructive operations are performed in dead fetuses to overcome pelvic contraction (as in craniotomy) or malpresentations (as in decapitation) following neglected labour.

The alternative would be to deliver these dead babies (following neglected labour) by cesarean section and exposing the mother to severe postoperative morbidity or death due to peritonitis, ileus and septic shock.

Incidence

The incidence depends on perinatal and transport services in a community. In developing countries of Asia and Africa it varies from 0.5 per cent to 1 per cent.

The types of destructive operations considered here are craniotomy, decapitation and craniocentesis as in hydrocephalus.

Craniotomy

This is the commonest destructive operation in obstetric practice in developing countries (Fig 10.5).

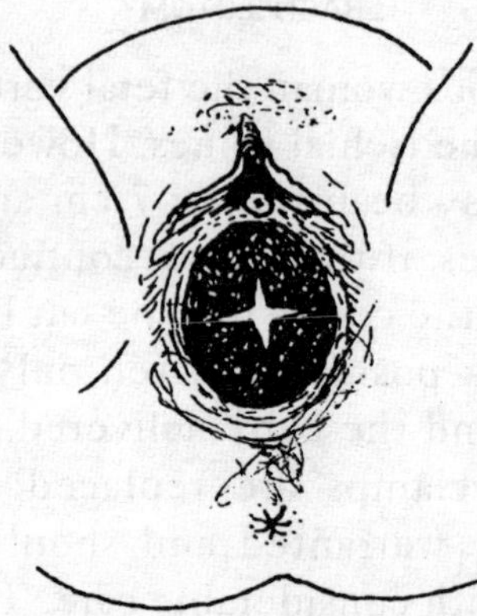

Fig 10.5 Cruciate incision on scalp for craniotomy

Case Report 1

A 27-year-old unbooked gravida 3, para 2 with previous normal deliveries (both are alive and the youngest child is 3 years old) is in full term labour for 20 hours. She was admitted for 'lack of progress in spite of good pains'. On examination she appeared exhausted, not anemic. Temp 38.5°C, pulse 104/min; BP 120/80 and Hb 10 g%. Abdominal examination showed the uterus contracting well with a Bandl's ring just below the umbilicus; head 2/5th felt; no FH audible. Per vaginum examination showed cervix fully dilated, head at station –2 with good degree of moulding and a large caput. After rapidly correcting dehydration and giving her IV antibiotics (chapter 18), an axis traction forceps was applied under anesthesia to steady the head. The fetal skull was then perforated with a Simpson's perforator passing it into the cranial cavity up to the shoulders of its blades before opening them. The blades were then closed and turned through 90 degrees and opened again to make a cruciform incision when the brain matter was seen coming out. Traction with forceps resulted in further compression with escape of more cranial contents. The head could now be easily delivered by forceps and the perforator was removed at the outlet as delivery of a dead female child (3.8 kg) was completed by forceps. Prophylactic oxytocics were given as soon as the anterior shoulders were born. There was no PPH. ***Comments:*** In this case of obstructed labour craniotomy was the preferred way. After the delivery, the bladder was drained for a week. Antibiotics were given for 6 more days. Lactation was suppressed with bromocryptine 2.5 mg tds orally for 5 days.

In mentoposterior position, in an impacted face presentation, perforation is done through orbit or palate after fixing it with an axis traction forceps. In the case of a breech the after-coming head is fixed by gentle traction on the trunk and the suboccipital region is perforated.

Decapitation

It is indicated in cases of neglected transverse lie, hand prolapse and dead fetus.

Case Report 2

8 am: A 32-year-old unbooked gravida 4, para 3 with spontaneous deliveries earlier (all alive, youngest child 2 years old) was admitted with history of labour pains (at 9th month) since midnight. The pains were sluggish till 3.30 am when she ruptured the membranes. An untrained midwife performed an internal examination and said that she felt the baby's hand in the vagina, and tried to push it in vain as the painful contractions became more frequent and stronger. Due to lack of transport she could not come earlier but reached the hospital 3 hours later.

On arrival, she looked dehydrated, not anemic, pulse 108/min; BP 110/70. The uterus appeared stretched transversely, with the possibility of the head on the right side. She had good uterine contractions, the lower segment was tender and fetal heart sounds were not heard. The prolapsed right arm appeared edematous and bluish. Per vaginum examination showed that the cervix was fully dilated.

Shoulder presentation was confirmed. After correcting dehydration rapidly and giving her prophylactic antibiotics IV she was anesthetised. Traction was applied on the prolapsed hand to make the neck more accessible. A decapitating hook was then carefully passed up to the fetal neck. Once it was firmly placed against the fetal neck, the handle of the decapitating hook was twisted to dislocate the neck. The embryotomy scissors were now used to cut the soft tissues of the neck. With continued traction on the prolapsed arm the headless fetal trunk was delivered. The head was delivered by suprapubic pressure and a finger in the child's mouth. (Alternatively, a volsellum can be applied to it and pulled out.) After the placenta was removed, the uterus was explored to rule out any tear. Prophylactic oxytocin was given to prevent PPH. She was discharged 5 days later.

Comments: In this case of neglected hand prolapse with a dead baby, decapitation was a suitable option. At the onset of labour if she had sought skilled care, an external cephalic version, failing which a cesarean section with tubal ligation, could have been done.

Evisceration

It is indicated in neglected transverse lie when the neck is not accessible. In this procedure, under anesthesia, after opening the fetal abdomen, evisceration followed by spondylotomy is performed and the fetus is delivered in two halves. In fetal ascites, the abdomen is deflated with sharp scissors or a perforator and then allowed to deliver. In a cephalic presentation with fetal ascites, abdominal paracentesis can be performed allowing vaginal delivery.

All cases of destructive operations require considerable skill and experience (more than for cesarean section). In these cases PPH and infection have to be prevented and the bladder drained for a week after the delivery to prevent bladder fistulas.

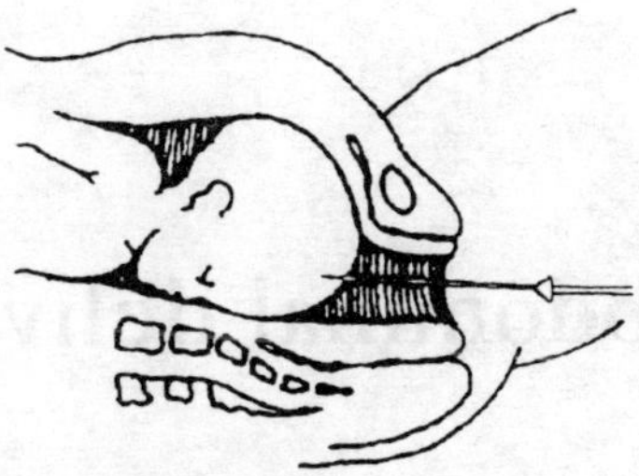

Fig 10.6 Craniocentesis

In developing countries, since there are still many cases of neglected labour, there is a need to train residents in these procedures. The alternative is cesarean section (with its attendant maternal risks).

Craniocentesis

In hydrocephalus at the pelvic brim, craniocentesis is performed in early labour with a wide bore needle or a perforator and vaginal delivery allowed (Fig 10.6). In breech, it could be done per abdomen under ultrasonographic guidance and local anesthesia. If delivered outside up to the neck, perforation or spinal tap is helpful.

Bibliography

Bofill JA, Brewit OA, Perry KG et al 1996. Forceps and vacuum delivery *Obstet Gynecol* 87: 1007–10.

Gibb DMF 1996. Operative Delivery. In: S Arulkumaran, SS Ratnam, KB Rao (Eds) *The Management of Labour.* Chennai: Orient Longman, 132–156.

Johnstone FD and Myerscough P R 1998. Shoulder dystocia. *Br J Obstet Gynecol* 105: 811–15.

Wong MT, Chua S and Arulkumaran S 1999. Operative vaginal delivery. In SS Ratnam, KB Rao and S Arulkumaran (Eds) *Obstetrics and Gynecology for Postgraduates* Vol 1, 2nd edn. Chennai: Orient Longman, 183–191.

11. Abdominal delivery

Abdominal delivery or cesarean section (CS) becomes necessary when safe vaginal delivery of a healthy child is not possible.

Incidence

Incidence varies but in a general population it should not be more than 14–15 per cent. Compared to the USA and Canada where the CS rate is over 20 per cent, it is less than 2 per cent in the sub-Saharan Africa.

Types of cesarean section

1. Lower uterine segment cesarean section (LSCS): This is the most common.
2. Classic or upper uterine segment CS: This is extremely rare.
3. Cesarean hysterectomy has a limited place and will be discussed later.

Classic cesarean section is associated with increased morbidity. Further, there is also (in a subsequent pregnancy) an increased risk of scar rupture (15–20 times higher than in LSCS). Therefore, the classic operation is rarely done these days without concurrent sterilisation.

Lower uterine segment cesarean section

Indications

Till a few decades ago, the indications were limited mostly

to pelvic dystocia, malpresentations like shoulder presentation, fetal distress and major degrees of placenta previa. However, due to advances in anesthesia, neonatology, and availability of blood transfusion and antibiotics there has been liberalisation of indications for CS.

The important indications at present are:

1. Dystocia due to a) passages – contracted pelvis, b) passenger – large baby, genuine CPD or due to malposition, c) forces – as in hypotonic inertia not responding to oxytocin infusion, d) malpresentations – breech, persistent mento-posterior, brow and shoulder
2. Repeat CS with recurrent indications (chapter 12)
3. Antepartum hemorrhage: most cases of placenta previa and 45–50 per cent of abruptio placentae cases (chapter 5)
4. Severe cases of PIH/eclampsia not responding to conservative therapy (chapter 4)
5. Fetal distress where immediate vaginal delivery is not possible (chapter 7).
6. Failed induction of labour associated with poor cervical score and the method used (Appendix 2)
7. Placental insufficiency as in prolonged pregnancy, elderly primipara, previous IUD, diabetes, cases of Rh isoimmunisation.
8. Bad obstetric history
9. Selected cases of multiple pregnancies (chapter 8)
10. Surgery on the reproductive tract as in cicatrised cervix after prolapse operations, or successful repair of urinary incontinence.
11. Patient's choice. However, this is not an ethical indication.

Anesthesia could be local, regional (spinal, epidural) or general (endotracheal intubation and ventilation with nitrous oxide, oxygen after giving relaxants) (chapter 19).

Procedure

Abdomen is opened with a right paramedian incision or a

Pfannenstiel incision. The peritoneum is opened with care not to injure the bladder. A bladder retractor is now placed over the pubic bone, the uterovesical peritoneal fold is picked up and incised transversely to push down the bladder and expose the lower uterine segment. The retractor should now retract the bladder (Fig 11.1). A transverse incision (2 cm long) is made with a scalpel in the lower segment (about 2 cm below the level of anterior peritoneal reflection or close to the leading edge of fetal head). The incision is now widened, by hooking a finger each at the edges of the incision, and pulling laterally and upwards. It is further incised gently and the bulging membranes are also incised. The hand is now inserted below the fetal head to lever it out (if necessary by applying fundal pressure simultaneously) (Fig 11.2). As soon as the head is delivered, the mucus is sucked out of the baby's mouth and the rest of the child is delivered

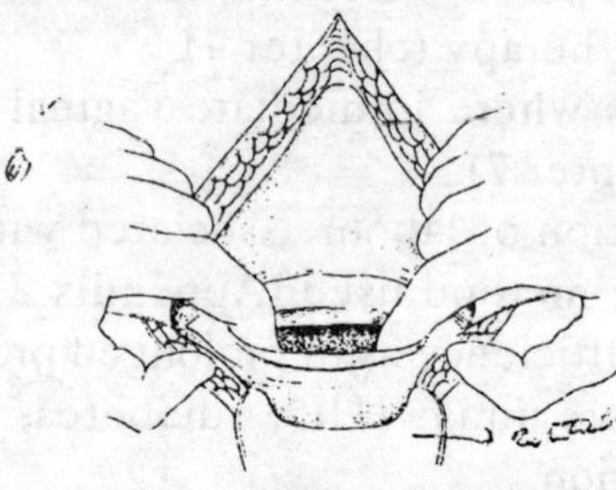

Fig 11.1 Bladder retractor

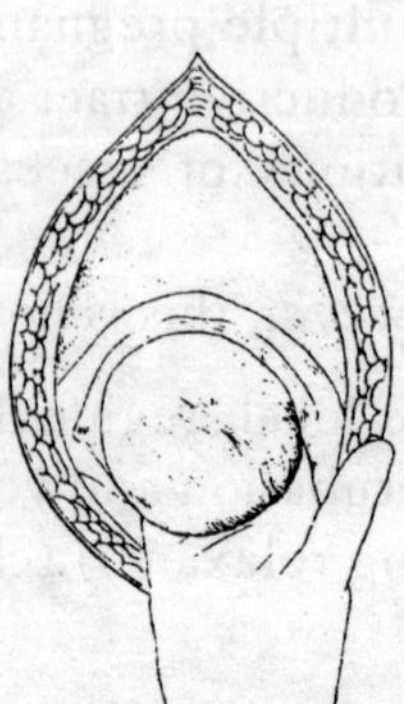

Fig 11.2 Delivering the baby's head

slowly. Oxytocin 20 units are now added to the saline drip and allowed to flow at 60 drops a minute. After the cord is clamped IV antibiotic (cefazolin 1 g or ampicillin 2 g) is given to the mother. After removal of the placenta and membranes a finger is passed through the cervical os. The uterine incision is sutured with continuous interlocking suture using No. 0 chromic catgut or vicryl. To obtain hemostasis and for better approximation, a second layer of suture is used. There is emerging evidence that single layer closure has a greater risk of scar dehiscence. The bleeders are arrested with a figure of eight stitch. After peritoneal toilet the abdomen is closed as it is not necessary to peritonise the lower segment.

Complications

The common complications of the surgery are

1. Postpartum hemorrhage
2. Difficulty in delivery of the head
3. Extension of the lower segment incision into the uterine artery
4. Injury to the bladder
5. Infection

Of these the commonest and the most serious is PPH. It is preventable by timely use of oxytocics. In addition to oxytocin drip, ergometrine 0.2 mg IV and/or carboprost 0.25 mg IM can be given; the latter could be repeated if necessary 10 minutes later. If atonic PPH is not controlled by bimanual compression of the uterus and oxytocics, ligation of uterine arteries is tried. In most cases, by this time, the bleeding is arrested. Vertical compression sutures where a catgut is passed from the anterior to the posterior wall in the lower segment and is brought upwards and tied at the fundus on either side has been shown to be simple and effective. In rare cases a subtotal hysterectomy is the only way to save the patient (chapter 10). In all cases of PPH, shock is treated (chapter 15).

Sometimes there may be some difficulty in delivering the head when it is fairly deep down in the pelvis and needs to be pushed up gently by an assistant to help it out. An alternative method would be to deliver the baby as a breech as the body flexes and comes out with ease while the head enters into the incision and is delivered.

Lateral extension of the incision may take place either initially when the lower segment wound is stretched by fingers or while delivering the baby's head or shoulders in haste. However, such extensions have to be sutured. The uterus gets its blood supply from two arteries and ligation of one does not have any negative effects provided the ureter is not included in the suture.

In case of bladder injury, its margins are mobilised and sutured with continuous interlocking sutures in two layers with No. 0 chromic catgut or vicryl taking care not to include the bladder mucosa while suturing. The bladder is continuously drained for 8 days.

Indications for a classic cesarean section

This is indicated in the following conditions either when the LSCS is not possible or is contraindicated:

1. Carcinoma cervix complicating pregnancy
2. When the lower segment is not accessible due to dense adhesions caused by previous surgery or pathology as in endometriosis.
3. Very vascular anterior lower segment as in some cases of placenta previa
4. A large myoma in the lower segment
5. Transverse lie in late labour

Procedure

Anesthesia is the same as for LSCS. An incision is made along the right paramedian. On opening the peritoneal cavity the uterus is brought to the midline and a vertical median incision about 9–10 cm long is made in the upper part of the uterus taking care that it stops short of the uterovesical peritoneal fold. The incision is extended deeper through the myometrium till the bulging membranes are seen. If the placenta is encountered it should be displaced laterally as cutting through it is difficult and can exsaguinate the fetus even with slight delay. The membranes are ruptured and the child is grasped at the ankle and extracted as in breech. After the cord is clamped oxytocics are administered (as described in LSCS). The uterine wound is closed in two layers of No. 0 chromic catgut or vicryl to ensure hemostasis. Bilateral tubal ligation is carried out (prior consent should have been taken) and the abdomen is closed in layers.

The important complications are:

1. PPH (managed as stated under LSCS).
2. The risk of scar rupture in the next pregnancy is prevented by sterilising the patient with her consent.
3. Scar endometriosis

Prognosis

One should not resort to a cesarean section unless it is indicated, since the maternal mortality is 5–7 times higher as compared to vaginal delivery. In addition she is exposed to further risks if she plans to have another pregnancy. No significant decrease in perinatal mortality is reported from institutions with higher CS rates.

HYSTERECTOMY

Obstetric hysterectomy is often subtotal as it is done as an emergency and time is of essence; also in most of these cases the cervix is healthy. However, in selected cases, the cervix or lower segment also require removal and total hysterectomy is done.

Indications

1. Uncontrollable PPH
2. Placenta previa accreta in a case of previous CS
3. Rupture uterus where rent cannot be repaired (chapter 7)
4. In a parous woman with symptomatic myomata when CS is done.

5. Following CS in case of gross intrapartum sepsis in a multipara.

Procedure

Anesthesia (preferably general) is given. The incision is subumbilical; median for postpartum hysterectomy but can be Pfannenstiel. The rest of the procedure is the same as for CS.

Subtotal hysterectomy: If during the course of a CS, a decision is made to do hysterectomy (due to intractable PPH) two clamps are applied to the round ligaments on either side and cut. The isthmic portion of the tubes and the ovarian ligaments too are similarly cut between clamps. The leaves of the broad ligament on either side are separated. The cesarean wound in the uterus is now clamped at the edges to include the uterine vessels. After these are securely ligated (with chromic No. 1 catgut), the incision is extended posteriorly and the uterus removed. The other clamps are now replaced by chromic catgut ligatures, which are transfixed and tied. Finally, the cervical stump is closed with figure of eight or interrupted chromic catgut sutures. After checking for hemostasis, the abdomen is closed in layers. She is treated for shock and given prophylactic antibiotics.

When a decision is made postpartum, the steps are similar except that the bladder has to be pushed down (after cutting the uterovesical fold of the peritoneum) as soon as the uterus is released from its lateral attachments till the base of broad ligaments. The clamps are then applied on either side close to the uterus to catch the uterine arteries and the supracervical portion of the uterus is now removed. The clamps are replaced with sutures and finally the cervical stump is closed as described earlier (Fig 11.3).

Total hysterectomy: This is necessary in a) colporrhexis or rupture involving the vaginal fornix, b) incomplete rupture of lateral uterine wall with broad ligament hematoma, c) placenta previa accreta with placenta in lower segment which has to be removed.

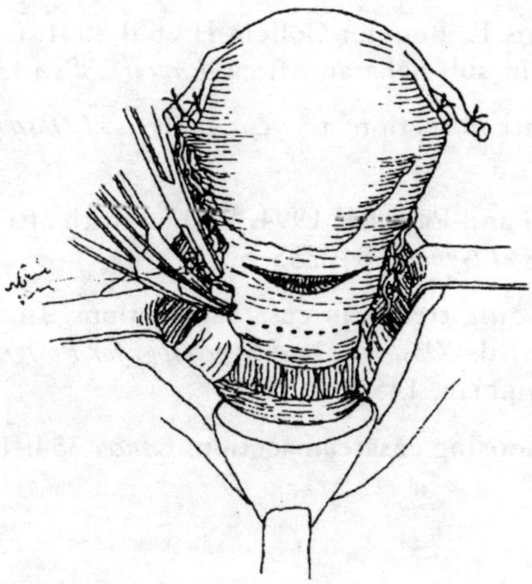

Fig 11.3 Subtotal hysterectomy

In a lateral tear (which usually occurs on the left side) left salpingo-oophorectomy may be required to treat the hematoma and catch the retracted cut lower end of uterine artery. To remove the cervix along with the uterus, it is necessary to push down the bladder to below the level of the cervix till the vaginal vault is reached. The next step is to clamp and cut the uterine artery on either side of the internal os close to the uterus (taking care to avoid injury to ureter). Straight clamps are now applied close to the uterus on either side to cut the Mackenrodt's ligaments. The uterosacrals are also cut posteriorly before opening the vaginal vault. The vagina is cut close to the cervix all round and the uterus is removed. After closure of the vaginal vault and checking for hemostasis the abdomen is closed in layers.

Complications

Complications are:

1. Hemorrhage
2. Injury to the ureter
3. Injury to the bladder

Bibliography

Dumont A, de Bernis L, Bouvier-Collem H et al 2001. Cesarean rate for maternal indication in sub-Saharan Africa. *Lancet* 358: 1328–34.

Kamala J 1995. Cesarean section: a 5 year analysis. *J Obstet Gynecol Ind* 49: 57–59.

Miller DA, Diaz FG and Paul RE 1994. Vaginal birth after cesarean: a 10 year experience. *Obstet Gynecol* 84: 255–58.

Rao KB 1999. Changing trends in cesarean sections. In SS Ratnam, KB Rao, S Arulkumaran (Eds) *Obstetrics and Gynecology for Postgraduates*. 2nd edn. Chennai: Orient Longman, 145–152.

Wagner M 2000. Choosing cesarean section. *Lancet* 354: 1677–80

12. Delivery following surgery on the reproductive tract

Labour following surgery on the reproductive tract needs tertiary care by a specialist to get the optimum result. The desire for good outcome has resulted in increasing cesarean section rates. With advancing technology more women are seen with operative scars in the reproductive tract. In this chapter we will discuss delivery following surgery on the uterus, cervix and vagina.

UTERUS

Surgery on the uterus may need to be performed for various reasons: cesarean section (lower segment and upper segment), myomectomy or corrective surgery for congenital anomalies of the uterus.

CESAREAN SECTION

This constitutes the largest group. Cesarean sections can be in the lower segment or (rarely) in the upper segment (classic cesarean section). Hysterotomy is rare in current practice but if it had been done, the case should be managed like a classic section. Cesarean section rates have been rising worldwide. In the West, CS rates vary between 15 and 25 per cent. Approximately 10 per cent of the obstetric population have been previously delivered by cesarean section. One in ten pregnant women and their care providers have to consider the risks and benefits of vaginal delivery against repeat elective cesarean section. The incidence of the rupture of the lower segment scar is approximately 3–5 per 1000 and that of classic ones are five to ten times higher. Recent literature based on a study of over 20,000 women with a previous cesarean scar suggests a rupture rate of 5 per 1000 in women with spontaneous labour, 8 per 1000 in women who had oxytocin and 25 per 1000 in women who had prostaglandins.

Selection of cases

The most dreaded complication while attempting vaginal delivery after cesarean section is the rupture of the scar. Therefore trial for vaginal delivery should be undertaken in places where appropriate facilities (for emergency cesarean section and blood transfusion) and personnel (midwife, anesthetic, obstetric and other support group staff) are available. If these facilities are not available it is wise not to have a trial or to transfer the women to a place where these facilities are available.

In these cases proper counselling of the woman and her partner is very important. They should be informed about the risks and benefits and an **informed consent** for trial for vaginal delivery will reflect good medical practice.

Favourable factors for successful labour and vaginal delivery are:

- Vaginal delivery before and after previous cesarean sections
- Cesarean sections done for non-recurrent causes, e.g. fetal distress
- The timing of the previous section in labour is an important guide to the type of uterine strain and work required in the next pregnancy. Women with previous CS in the active phase of labour (cervix fully effaced and cervix > 3 cm dilation) usually show a multiparous pattern of labour with less uterine work, whereas women who have a CS in the latent phase of labour or with no

labour will show greater uterine activity (more than multiparas but less than nulliparas).

- In cases of dystocia being the cause of previous section, the chance of successful vaginal delivery is slightly reduced but if there are no other contraindications, vaginal delivery may be attempted.
- Preliminary studies suggest that ultrasonographic and magnetic resonance imaging measurement of the lower uterine segment may help select those with a higher risk of scar rupture. Their use has not been properly validated in clinical practice and more studies are needed in this area.

Unfavourable factors are:

- Any uterine scar that encroaches on the upper uterine segment is a contraindication. This includes classic cesarean section, hysterotomy and many cases of low vertical cesarean section where incision often encroaches on the upper uterine segment. Inverted T type incisions make weak scars and are best not subjected to labour.
- Cases with two or more previous lower segment cesarean section have a slightly increased chance of scar rupture. There have been few reports in the literature of successful delivery following two lower segment cesarean sections.
- Previous uterine rupture is a contraindication.
- Other obstetric complications such as placenta previa or transverse lie. In twin pregnancy overdistension of the uterus may cause a problem in rare cases. Intrauterine manipulation for delivery of the second twin increases the potential risk of uterine rupture.
- Individual factors such as maternal age, history of subfertility and previous perinatal loss
- The woman must be informed and committed. Coercion, subtle or otherwise is inappropriate.

In each case an appropriate decision has to be made on the merits of the case.

Management

Antenatal care: Apart from a detailed review of the factors listed above, antenatal care should be routine and a decision should be made for the type of delivery after proper counselling and discussion with the patients. Post-cesarean cases are high-risk cases; at antenatal visits enquire specifically about suprapubic pain or vaginal bleeding.

Induction of labour: As with other cases for induction of labour there should be a valid reason for induction of labour in post-cesarean cases; if the cervix is favourable, amniotomy is the method of choice. This may be followed by careful administration of oxytocin if needed but **labour** has to be **monitored very closely**. Uterine activity profiles after augmentations in post-cesarean cases have shown increase in frequency, amplitude and uterine strength. The rate of progress in the first 3–4 hours after augmentation appears to indicate the outcome. In cases of unfavourable cervix prostaglandins may be used. A number of reviews mainly from tertiary hospitals suggest that judicious use of oxytocin and prostaglandins for cervical ripening and induction of labour is reasonable in women with one previous transverse lower segment cesarean section. However such practice increases the risk of scar dehiscence or rupture and the woman should be informed about it.

Labour: The woman who has had a previous cesarean section should be advised to come into hospital early in labour. If the fetus is in the longitudinal lie and the head fixed to the pelvic brim and there is no scar pain or tenderness she could be allowed to ambulate. Once labour has been established it is preferable to have an intravenous line and blood should be sent for grouping and typing. Continuous electronic fetal heart monitoring (EFM) is not routinely done in early labour. It is beneficial in active labour as one of the earliest signs of uterine dehiscence is abnormality of the fetal heart rate. Epidural analgesia may be provided for pain relief as indicated for any other labour. The theoretical risk of masking uterine rupture pain has not been substantiated.

The progress of labour should be carefully charted using a partogram. In non-progressive labour oxytocin augmentation may be considered but only in hospitals with on site obstetric and anesthetic personnel. If augmentation is undertaken, a smooth progressive response should be observed and if this does not occur a repeat cesarean section should be performed. The patient is watched carefully for signs and symptoms of early uterine rupture and they include:

1. Persistent pain and tenderness over the lower uterine segment between uterine contractions
2. Fetal heart rate abnormality is the most consistent and reliable early warning sign, although it is not specific to scar rupture. This may include tachycardia, prolonged late and variable decelerations or persistent bradycardia, the latter being the most worrying sign.
3. Vaginal bleeding
4. The bladder is often adherent to the site of a lower segment scar and hematuria may be one of the early signs if the integrity of the scar and adherent bladder is disrupted.
5. Maternal hypotension, tachycardia and syncope
6. Disengagement and displacement of the fetal head. In thin women a unilateral swelling over the lower uterine segment may be detected.

The lower segment scar is thin, relatively avascular, and may dehisce with minimal clinical signs. A catastrophic picture of sudden severe lower abdominal pain, vaginal bleeding, cessation of uterine contractions, fetal death and signs of intra-abdominal hemorrhage are fortunately rare with rupture of previous low transverse cesarean scars.

In many hospitals about 50–60 per cent women may be expected to deliver safely vaginally after previous cesarean section. However, no large randomised studies have compared trial of vaginal delivery with elective cesarean section. A meta-analysis of studies from the last decade suggests a slightly increased risk of the rare event of uterine rupture and neonatal morbidity and mortality with a trial for vaginal delivery and an increased rate of maternal morbidity with elective cesarean section.

With careful selection the majority of women will have a smooth and progressive labour, achieving vaginal delivery with minimal risk to the mother and the infant. When additional risk factors are present, the risk of scar rupture increases with very little gain in the number of vaginal deliveries. Excessive zeal in trying to achieve a vaginal delivery leads to unreasonable risk and this is another area in clinical medicine where sensible clinical judgement is required.

Myomectomy

Women with previous history of myomectomy should be treated like those who have had cesarean section. In the majority of cases the fibroids are in the body of the uterus, that is, in the upper segment. It has been advocated that if the endometrium has been breached during myomectomy, elective cesarean section is preferred due to a weak scar. Whether the endometrium has been breached or not, each case has to be decided on its merit, associated factors involved, such as history of subfertility, miscarriages, bad obstetric history and patient's wish after proper counselling should be taken into account. If vaginal delivery has been tried, the patient should be closely monitored.

Operations on the Cervix

Cervical cytological screening has reduced the incidence of invasive carcinoma of the cervix. However, in view of the abnormal cervical smear and colposcopic findings many childbearing women undergo treatment by loop excision of the transformation zone, laser vaporisation or cold knife cone biopsy.

Cold knife cone biopsy has been associated with preterm labour but it depends on the size of the cone. It has been noted that the larger the size of the cone the greater is the incidence of preterm labour and simple cervical cerclage does not appear to reduce the risk of preterm labour following cone biopsy. In rare cases, cone biopsy may be associated with cervical stenosis and non-dilatation of the cervix in labour. The complication rates following laser surgery or loop excision have been found to be much less than with knife cone biopsy; it is also not very different from that seen in the general population.

Recently conservative operation for early carcinoma of cervix (radical trachelotomy) has been tried with a view that the childbearing function can be maintained. High incidence of preterm labour and mid-trimester pregnancy loss has been reported in animal studies and this group will probably require prophylactic abdominal cerclage operations. The efficacy and results of this operation are still being evaluated. In cases of Manchester operation, cervical elongation has been performed, there is a risk of preterm labour or cervical stenosis in labour depending on the length of cervix that has been amputated.

Operations for Correction of Congenital Anomalies

Operations done for the correction of congenital anomalies may influence the outcome of pregnancy and delivery. A rudimentary horn of uterus should be resected before the woman starts her obstetric career as the outcome of a ruptured pregnant horn can be potentially fatal to the mother and the fetus. For future pregnancies cesarean section is desirable if the endometrial cavity of the other horn has been entered during the resection of the rudimentary horn.

Hysteroscopic resection of the uterine septae or submucous fibroid is usually not related with delivery problems. However, increased incidence of placental non-separation in the third stage has been reported.

Miscellaneous Operations

Other operations on the reproductive tract include anterior

colporrhaphy, operations for stress incontinence, Manchester repair and repair of fourth degree tears. These are reconstructive operations and ideally these operations, apart from repair of fourth degree tear, should be done after completion of childbearing functions. In pregnant women with a history of these operations elective cesarean section should be performed to prevent injury to the repaired tissues. Vaginal delivery may be attempted in women with a history of previous third degree tear. An experienced obstetrician should be present during the second stage and all measures should be taken to prevent recurrence of a tear. Some studies have shown more sphincter damage after vaginal birth; offering an elective cesarean section is a reasonable option in these cases.

Women who are pregnant following operations on the reproductive tract should be treated as high-risk patients. Each case has to be decided on its own merit and decisions regarding the mode of delivery are to be made after taking all relevant factors into consideration and with the informed consent of the woman.

Bibliography

Arulkumaran S, Chua S and Ratnam SS 1992. Symptoms and signs in scar dehiscence. *Austr NZ Obstet Gynecol* 20:

Chua S, Arulkumaran S and Ratnam SS 1996. Pregnancy following cesarean section. In: SS Ratnam, S Arulkumaran and KB Rao (Eds) *Management of Labour.* Chennai: Orient Longman, 317–27.

Duhurst CJ 1957. Previous cesarean scar rupture. *J Obstet Gynecol Br C'wlth* 64: 117–118.

Goldbert AB, Genless MB and Dany PD 2001. Misoprostol in pregnancy. *N Engl J Med* 344: 38–47.

Kurian J 2003. Uterine prolapse. In SS Ratnam, KB Rao and S Arulkumaran (Eds) *Obstetrics and Gynecology for Postgraduates* Vol. 2, 2nd edn. Chennai: Orient Longman.

Sultan MM 1993. Anal sphincter rupture after vaginal delivery. *N Engl J Med* 329: 1905–11.

Zelop CM, Shipp TD, Repke JT et al 2000. Effect of previous vaginal delivery on the risk of uterus rupture during a subsequent trial of labour. *Am J Obstet Gynecol*, 183(5):1184-86.

13. Medical emergencies in obstetrics

HEART DISEASE IN PREGNANCY

Incidence

Incidence is 0.5–1 per cent of pregnant women.

Etiology

In 80 per cent of women, these are due to acquired causes and in 20 per cent it is congenital. The most common acquired lesion is rheumatic mitral valve disease. Septal defects and patent ductus are the predominant congenital lesions. Cyanotic congenital valvular disorders like Fallot's tetralogy are rare.

The cardiovascular changes occurring in normal pregnancy increases the work load on the heart. Blood volume increases by 40 per cent, the pulse rate by 10 beats/min and the cardiac output by 30 per cent. There is decreased peripheral resistance. These changes are gradual, starting from early pregnancy and reaching a peak in early third trimester and in the peripartum period. A diseased heart which is not able to withstand this extra strain may fail early or during periods of peak cardiac output.

Signs and symptoms and diagnosis

These depend on the type and duration of cardiac lesion, the period of gestation and the response to effort. They may vary from palpitation and tachycardia to cyanosis, dyspnea, pedal edema, tender enlarged liver and coarse rales in both the lungs.

Depending on the response to effort, a pregnant woman with cardiac disease may be classified as belonging to one of the following classes (New York Heart Association):

Class 1: Cardiac lesion with no restriction of normal activity.
Class 2: Slight restriction with breathlessness at the end of normal activity.
Class 3: Moderate restriction; slightest effort ends in dyspnea.
Class 4: Dyspnea even at rest.

On clinical examination the apex beat may be felt beyond the midclavicular line with a presystolic thrill and a murmur in mitral stenosis. In case of doubt, echocardiography is extremely useful.

Prognosis and complications

The complications are:

- Acute pulmonary edema which has a worse outlook than congestive heart failure. Pulmonary hypertension, respiratory infections, anemia and PIH may precipitate heart failure.
- Atrial fibrillation may cause failure and/or thromboembolism.

Maternal mortality is about 5 per cent in grade 4 cases. In Eisenmenger's syndrome (pulmonary hypertension with a left to right shunt) it is over 40 per cent, and in peripartum cardiomyopathy it is 20 per cent. Perinatal mortality is 10 per cent and is mainly due to prematurity.

Management

All pregnant women with heart disease should be seen once a fortnight till 28 weeks and weekly thereafter till labour, jointly by the cardiologist and the obstetrician. She is advised about her diet, exercise, prevention of anemia and respiratory infections.

During labour she could adopt a position comfortable to her, and is given oxygen and digoxin when needed. The second stage is usually short, but in case of delay it is cut short by an outlet forceps under pudendal block. In the third stage, oxytocin is used but not ergometrine as it may raise the blood pressure. Generally, the indications for induction of labour and for cesarean section should be only for obstetric reasons and not because of the cardiac lesion. Prostaglandins are avoided in heart disease. For cesarean section, epidural or general anesthesia may be given.

Congestive cardiac failure is treated with:

- Rest in bed in semi-recumbent position; salt and fluid restriction
- Oxygen
- Sedation: morphine 10 mg IM
- Furosemide 40 mg IV
- Digoxin 0.25 mg tablet twice or thrice daily, depending on her pulse rate. In severe cases digoxin 0.5 mg may be needed IM followed by oral medication.

In atrial fibrillation, beta-blockers, digoxin and anticoagulants are required.

In acute pulmonary edema, rest, oxygen, furusemide 80 mg IV and morphine 2–3 mg IV are useful.

In case of mitral stenosis with a valve area less than 1 cm^2, balloon mitral valvotomy may be useful for continuation of pregnancy. Cardiovascular surgery if indicated is best done in early pregnancy as the risks are greater in late pregnancy and in early puerperium. In those with mitral valve replacement taking oral anticoagulants, heparin (preferably low molecular weight) is needed in the early weeks (to prevent teratogenicity) and again after 36 weeks. In early labour and postpartum prophylactic antibiotics may be useful. For contraception, the barrier method is advised as IUCD and combined oral pills are contraindicated.

ANEMIA IN PREGNANCY

Anemia in pregnancy is defined as pregnancy with hemoglobin (Hb) concentration of less than 10 g/dl or hematocrit (Hct) of less than 33 per cent.

Incidence

1. It is the commonest medical disorder in pregnancy and is seen in 75 per cent of pregnant women in South Asia. It may be mild (Hb 8.0–10.9 g%), moderate (Hb 5.0–7.9 g%) or severe (Hb < 5 g% or Hct < 24 per cent).

Etiology

1. The commonest cause is nutritional deficiency, usually of iron. Folate deficiency is rare, and is seen in multiple pregnancies and in areas endemic to malaria.
2. Parasitic infestations as in malaria and hookworm infestations.
3. Chronic infections as in pyelonephritis and AIDS.
4. In hemolytic anemias: Hemoglobinopathies like thalassemia and sickle cell disease.

For the increase in blood volume, growth of uterus, breasts, fetus and placenta during pregnancy, extra iron is needed. The daily requirement of iron is estimated to be less than 1 mg in early pregnancy, but goes up to 5 mg in the second trimester, and 8 mg in the last trimester. In most developing countries, the diet does not supply this iron. Thus in the absence of iron supplements a healthy woman may develop anemia or a preexisting anemic mother may become worse during pregnancy.

Signs, symptoms and diagnosis

Women with mild anemia may complain of fatigue; those with moderate to severe anemia may experience breathlessness and edema. There is pallor of the conjunctiva and tongue with flat or spoon-shaped nailbeds. A person with severe anemia may present a picture of congestive cardiac failure.

Diagnosis is confirmed from the estimation of Hb and Hct values, and examination of peripheral blood smear (mostly microcytic hypochromic; malarial parasite may also be seen in endemic areas). The blood smear and examination of stools may help to find the cause of anemia. Serum iron < 30 μg/dl and the total iron binding capacity (TIBC) of > 400 μg/dl are diagnostic of iron deficiency anemia.

Complications and prognosis

Complications are:

1. Congestive cardiac failure (especially when Hb is < 5 g per cent and pregnancy less than 20 weeks)
2. Premature labour
3. Infection
4. Thromboembolism in puerperium

Maternal mortality is 15 per cent in severe anemia. Anemia is the commonest cause of associated maternal deaths in developing countries.

Prevention

Oral iron (ferrous sulphate) and folic acid tablets (IFA) each with 60 mg of elemental iron and 0.5 mg of folic acid is recommended throughout pregnancy. As most adolescents and non-pregnant women are anemic (especially in malarial endemic areas), they are advised one IFA tablet daily. When examination of stools show hookworms, mebendazole 100 mg is given orally twice daily for 3 days except in the first trimester.

Management

In pregnancy: In mild cases 2 IFA tablets (120 mg elemental iron and 1 mg folate) are given orally daily till term. Deworming and antimalarials are administered when necessary.

In moderate cases, parenteral iron (IM iron is advised, because of risk of anaphylaxis when it is given IV), depending on the deficit. For example, if Hb is 6 g%, to bring it up to 12 g% she will need (12–6) x 2 x 85 mg or a total of 1020 mg to which 50 per cent more is added to replenish maternal stores. After a test dose of 50 mg of IM iron, she is administered 200 mg IM daily till the deficit is wiped out. She is monitored regularly till term.

In severe anemia, packed cell transfusion is given slowly preceded by furosemide 40 mg IV. Later she is given 2 tablets of IFA daily.

During labour: Most anemic women deliver prematurely and spontaneously. If there is any delay in the second stage, it should be cut short with an outlet forceps. PPH must be prevented at all costs by prophylactic oxytocics (including ergometrine) as blood loss of even 200 or 250 ml may produce shock. If she is admitted in labour with moderate to severe anemia, packed cell transfusion is given preceded by furosemide 40 mg IV as stated earlier.

After delivery she is advised oral iron for 2 months.

JAUNDICE IN PREGNANCY

Jaundice or yellowish discoloration of the conjunctiva is seen in about 0.5 per cent pregnancies in India. During outbreaks of viral hepatitis, jaundice in pregnancy carries much higher maternal and fetal risks.

Etiology

The most common cause in developing countries is viral hepatitis. The viruses often encountered are hepatitis E virus (HEV) and hepatitis A virus (HAV) due to contaminated water supply, the route of infection being feco-oral. Of the blood borne viruses (HBV, HCV, HDV), HBV is the commonest. Its transmission is through infected blood and its products, contaminated needles and by sexual intercourse. Rarer causes are cholestatic jaundice and use of hepatotoxic drugs.

In one series of 169 cases of viral hepatitis in pregnancy 82 per cent were due to HEV, 17 per cent due to HBV and only 1 per cent due to HAV.

Signs, symptoms and diagnosis

In the prodromal phase of infective hepatitis, the patient may have fever, vomiting and loss of appetite. A week later, the icteric phase follows when the conjunctiva is yellowish with passage of tea-coloured urine and clay-coloured stools. The liver may be tender and palpable. The urine contains bile pigments and bile salts. Serum bilirubin levels may even exceed 15 mg% and serum may later show viral antibodies. The jaundice may last for 10–14 days.

Complications and prognosis

Fulminant hepatitis and hepatic failure are possible complications. If hepatitis rapidly progresses she becomes drowsy followed by coma and convulsions often ending in a premature delivery with PPH (due to prothrombin deficiency) and death. It is usually seen in the last trimester of pregnancy and carries a maternal mortality of 20 per cent and perinatal mortality of 30–50 per cent.

Treatment

Treatment is mainly preventive–protected water supply, use of sterile needles and safe blood. Vaccination against HAV is advised in an endemic area. All persons testing negative for HBsAg should be vaccinated with a recombinant vaccine against HBV. All newborns should be protected with a recombinant vaccine against HBV (10 mg at birth, 1, 3 and 12 months of pregnancy). If the mother is HBeAg+ the newborn is given 0.5 ml HBIg in addition to the vaccine.

Curative therapy is on the same general lines as in the non-pregnant person with bedrest, high calorie diet and oral neomycin. If vomiting is present she is given IV dextrose solution.

In viral hepatitis there is no place for termination of pregnancy or induction. Surgery should only be performed if it is absolutely unavoidable. PPH must be prevented and if coagulation failure occurs, it is appropriately treated (chapter 5). In hepatic failure the prognosis is grave.

Cholestatic jaundice is usually mild and obstructive. It often recurs in successive pregnancies. Apart from itching and a risk of premature delivery, there is a slightly increased risk of perinatal death and may warrant induction of labour.

RENAL DISEASE IN PREGNANCY

In normal pregnancy there is an increase in the renal plasma flow and in glomerular filtration pressure leading to a rise in the GFR and creatinine clearance. In patients with underlying renal disease and hypertension, the BP goes up further during pregnancy. If there is superimposed preeclampsia the endothelial injury poses a challenge to their management. Thus, in cases of renal disease it is necessary to assess preconceptional renal function and counsel the patient about the risks. If preconceptional serum creatinine is below 1.5 mg% the prognosis is considered favourable.

It is possible to have a successful pregnancy following renal transplantation after at least 2 years of normal functioning of the transplanted kidney in a woman who is normotensive and is on minimal doses of immuno-suppressants. She requires careful monitoring as 50 per cent of such women may deliver prematurely. The chances of rejection are 10 per cent and there is deterioration of renal function in 15 per cent following a pregnancy.

Acute Pyelonephritis in Pregnancy

Urinary tract infections are ten times more common in women than in men. It is commoner in the pregnant woman.

Incidence

Incidence is about 2 per cent of pregnancies.

Etiology

Urine is a good culture medium for bacterial growth. In pregnancy, dilatation of the ureter and renal pelvis lead to urinary stasis predisposing to infection. Asymptomatic bacilluria is seen in 5 per cent of pregnant women and if left untreated, 20 per cent will develop pyelonephritis. In 80 per cent of these the pathogen is E. coli. In those cases where infections are associated with a catheter or due to calculi, proteus and pseudomonas may be the causative pathogen.

Signs, symptoms and diagnosis

In mild cases she may have nausea, fever and dysuria. In severe cases, persistent vomiting, fever with rigor and loin pain may be present. Occasionally there may be hematuria. The diagnosis may be confirmed by presence of pyuria (>10 pus cells/high power field of a clean catch urine) and from the bacteriological growth on urine culture.

Differential diagnosis

1. Malaria
2. Acute appendicitis
3. Preeclampsia

Complications

Complications are premature labour, IUGR, recurrent pyelonephritis, endotoxic shock (when virulent strains are involved) and chronic renal disease.

Management

Preventive: Treatment of asymptomatic bacilluria based on latest culture and sensitivity report. This is usually with oral quinolones (oral ciprofloxacin 500 mg 12 hours for 7 days) or amoxycillin 500 mg 8 hourly for 7 days. Urine culture has to be repeated monthly till delivery.

In severe pyelonephritis, 5% dextrose saline IV may be needed till vomiting is controlled. Parenteral ciprofloxacin (400 mg 12 hourly) or ceftriaxone 1–2 g/day or gentamycin (1mg/kg/day) may be given till fever subsides. This is followed by oral quinolones or cephalosporins depending on the sensitivity report. When there is no response or in recurrent infections, ultrasonography may be needed to rule out any structural anomaly or obstructive uropathy. As all calculi cannot be detected by ultrasonography, a skiagram may be necessary.

Continuous low dose prophylaxis with nitrofurantoin may be needed in recurrent infections in pregnancy.

DIABETES COMPLICATING PREGNANCY

Diabetes is a metabolic disorder characterised by hyperglycemia, which may be due to reduced insulin production, decreased capacity for glucose storage or excess production of glucose.

Incidence

Incidence is about 5 per cent of all pregnant women.

Etiology

In Type 1 it is due to autoimmune beta-cell destruction of the pancreas. Type 2 diabetes is due to increased insulin resistance, impaired insulin secretion or increased glucose production. In gestational diabetes mellitus (GDM) impaired glucose tolerance (IGT) is seen early followed by increased insulin resistance and hyperglycemia. The risk factors for GDM are:

1. Family history of diabetes in parent or a sibling
2. Obesity
3. Previously identified IGT
4. Previous obstetric history of GDM, macrosomia, recurrent fetal deaths, PIH, and fetal anomaly

Signs, symptoms and diagnosis

Pregnancy is associated with marked insulin resistance and increased insulin requirement precipitating GDM. In early stages there are no typical symptoms. The diagnosis is made by screening for plasma glucose after an oral 50 g GTT between 24 and 28 weeks in all cases of glycosuria in pregnancy and in those with risk factors mentioned earlier. If the 1 hour post 50 g oral glucose challenge value is more than 140 mg/dl, 100 g oral glucose tolerance test is done (Table 13.2). If two or more threshold values are met or exceeded in the 100 g oral GTT, it is confirmatory of gestational diabetes (Expert Committee 2000).

In early pregnancy hyperglycemia acts as a teratogen. Later, it stimulates the fetal pancreas to produce excess of insulin, the anabolic effect of which is responsible for macrosomia. In GDM, there is increased incidence of hydramnios and hypertension (PIH) which may lead to IUGR, fetal hypoxia and its demise near term.

*Table 13.1 Criteria for diagnosis of diabetes in the non-pregnant**

	Normal	*Impaired glucose tolerance*	*Diabetes mellitus*
Fasting plasma glucose (mg per cent)	< 110 mg per cent (< 6.1 mmol/l)	110–120	> 126 (7.0 mmol/l)
2 h post 75 g oral glucose challenge	< 140 (7.8 mmol/l)	140–199	> 200 (> 11.1 mmol/l)

*Adapted from Report of the *Expert Committee on the Diagnosis and Classification of Diabetes Mellitus* (2000)

Table 13.2 Criteria for diagnosis of gestational diabetes

(Criteria require that 2 or more thresholds be exceeded)

Status	*Plasma glucose (mg/dl)*	*Plasma glucose (mmol/l)*
Fasting	105	5.8
One hour*	190	10.6
Two hours*	165	9.2
Three hours*	145	8.0

*100 g oral glucose tolerance test

Adapted from Report of the *Expert Committee on the Diagnosis and Classification of Diabetes Mellitus* (2000)

Complications and prognosis

Maternal:

Increased risk of

PIH

Infections of urinary tract and vaginal candidiasis

Diabetic ketosis in the presence of hyperemesis, infections or during labour.

Operative morbidity due to fetal macrosomia and PIH.

Perinatal:

Macrosomia

Prematurity

IUGR

Perinatal hypoxia and death

Neonatal:

RDS or pulmonary hyaline membrane disease, hypoglycemia, hypocalcemia and hyperbilirubinemia.

Perinatal mortality has declined from 15 per cent to less than 5 per cent after introduction of insulin and careful fetal monitoring.

Management

The aim is to maintain euglycemia from early pregnancy (to prevent fetal malformations and macrosomia), monitor fetal growth and deliver a live child near term. The goal is to maintain the blood sugar (HbA_{1c} below 7%) in the range 5.5–7.8 mmol/l or 100–140 mg% at bedtime and glycolated. Initially the control is achieved by regulation of diet (30 kcal/kg for non-obese women; for obese women caloric restriction not to exceed 30–33 per cent) and exercise. If necessary insulin (huminsulin) is to be used only if nutritional therapy has not resulted in fasting plasma glucose levels less than 95 mg/dl or 1 hour post-prandial values less than 130–140 mg/dl or 2 hours post-prandial values less than 120 mg/dl. Oral antidiabetic drugs should not be used during pregnancy.

These patients require to be seen at least once in two

weeks jointly with a diabetalogist. Ultrasonography is performed at 20 weeks and after 32 weeks, and as and when necessary to monitor growth. If PIH or IUGR are present, Doppler flow studies may also be required twice weekly. After 36 weeks more frequent monitoring with non-stress test helps in deciding the time and mode of delivery. Induction of labour is advised after 37 weeks if the cervix is ripe.

Cesarean section is indicated if there is:

1. Macrosomia (weight > 4.5 kg)
2. IUGR
3. Suspicion of antenatal fetal hypoxia (non-reactive NST or diminished fetal activity)
4. Fetal distress in labour as per CTG or meconium stained liquor
5. Previous bad obstetric history
6. Previous cesarean section for GDM
7. PIH not responding to therapy between 33 and 37 weeks (betamethasone to be given 24 hours prior to cesarean section (chapter 6)
8. The newborn has to be carefully looked after to prevent hypoxia, hypoglycemia (chapter 14).

After delivery the insulin dose has to be reduced or stopped. Infection has to be prevented and contraceptive advice offered.

If at any time ketosis occurs, it has to be promptly treated as an acute emergency. In these cases, plasma glucose values will be high; in addition, potassium, sodium, chlorine, bicarbonate and creatinine estimations are also required. Urinary output has to be monitored. In 1–3 hours she is given 2–3 litres of normal saline IV followed by 5% dextrose saline when plasma glucose level has come down to 250 mg%. Later 5–10 units of insulin is given by IV drip regulating the plasma glucose which is monitored hourly. In addition electrolytes, acid base balance, BP, pulse, urine output and mental status are also monitored. The goal is to maintain plasma glucose values between 150 and 250 mg%. Antibiotics are given to combat infection.

MALARIA COMPLICATING PREGNANCY

Malaria is widely prevalent in developing countries of Asia and Africa and is responsible for significant maternal morbidity and mortality.

Incidence

It is more common among young primigravidas rather than the older multiparous women even in the same area as the latter develop some immunity.

Etiology

The causative agent is a protozoan parasite plasmodium. The commonest is P. vivax. In certain areas P. falciparum and P ovale are seen. Transmission occurs when an infected female anopheles mosquito injects the sporozoites into a human host while sucking blood.

Signs, symptoms and diagnosis

Intermittent fever with rigor often associated with vomiting, headache and myalgia are common complaints. In falciparum infections, the disease may be more severe and the fever is accompanied by drowsiness, coma and convulsions. Cerebral malaria is often misdiagnosed as eclampsia. In chronic cases one may find hepatosplenomegaly.

The diagnosis is confirmed when a thick peripheral blood smear taken during the fever with rigor reveals parasites in the RBCs. In some laboratories more sensitive methods like the quick buffy coat (QBC), rapid antigen detection test or polymerase chain reaction (PCR) may be available. A smear from the placental surface soon after a premature delivery may also show the parasites as they accumulate there. Only in a rare case of very heavy parasitemia a few parasites may cross the placental barrier to cause congenital malaria.

Differential diagnosis

Differential diagnosis may be acute pyelonephritis or eclampsia.

Complications and prognosis

Complications are premature labour, IUGR and anemia. In falciparum infections, additional complications are cerebral malaria, severe anemia, shock, DIC, hemoglobinuria (black water fever), hyopoglycemia and pneumonia. In malaria generally the fatality rate is less than 0.5 per cent, but in cerebral malaria in pregnancy it is over 30 per cent.

Management

Preventive: Use of mosquito nets soaked in DDT solution and chemoprophylaxis. Certain antimalarials like doxycycline and primaquine (the latter may produce G6PD deficiency) are not considered safe in pregnancy. As safety information for use of Proguanil in pregnancy is insufficient, chloroquine 300 mg weekly orally is favoured. In areas where parasites are resistant to chloroquine, mefloquine 250 mg weekly orally is recommended.

Curative: In uncomplicated cases chloroquine is the drug of choice (10 mg/kg body weight) orally once daily for 2 days followed by 5 mg/kg on third day. However, in falciparum, areas 3 tablets of sulfadoxine + pyrimethamine (each consisting of sulfadoxine 500 mg + pyrimethamine 25 mg) have been used in some African countries for curative purposes in the seventh and eighth months of pregnancy leading to reduction of low birth weight and maternal mortality rates (WHO 2000a). In areas where the parasite is resistant to chloroquine, either quinine sulphate 10 mg/kg thrice daily orally for 7 days, or mefloquine 15 mg/kg on day 1 and 10 mg/kg on day 2 is preferred (WHO 2000a). Alternatively, artesunate is given as 4 mg/kg orally on day 1 followed by 2 mg/kg daily for the next 6 days (Table 13.3).

Severe and complicated malaria

As the patient may have persistent vomiting, 5% dextrose is given as IV drip followed by chloroquine injections; later chloroquine is given orally. In resistant areas and in cerebral malaria parenteral administration of quinine dichloride with

Table 13.3 Curative treatment of uncomplicated and complicated malaria

Antimalarial drug	*Uncomplicated malaria*	*Complicated malaria*
Chloroquine	(Oral) 10 mg/kg on days 1 and 2, followed by 5 mg/kg on day 3	10 mg/kg IV infusion over 8 h followed by 15 mg/kg IV over 24 h; or 3.5 mg/kg IM every 6 h
Mefloquine	15 mg/kg first dose followed by 10 mg/kg 24 h later	
Fansidar	Sulfadoxine 500 mg + Pyrimethamine / table	3 tablets
Quinine	10 mg/kg three times a day for 7 days	20 mg/kg IV infusion over 4 h followed by 10 mg/kg IV over 2–8 h every 8 h; later oral
Artesunate	4 mg/kg loading dose orally on day 1 followed by 2 mg/kg for 6 days	2.4 mg/kg IV followed by 1.2 mg/kg at 12 and 24 h and then daily till she regains consciousness
Artemether	—	3.2 mg/kg IM on day 1 followed by 1.6 mg/kg per day

a loading dose of 20 mg/kg followed by 10 mg/kg as maintenance dose is given till she regains consciousness. With oral medication, ensure that the patient completes 7 days of therapy. Alternatively, artemesinin derivatives could be given parenterally and later orally.

In complicated falciparum infections it will be necessary to monitor plasma glucose 6 hourly, Hct 8–12 hourly and creatinine daily, besides maintaining an intake and output chart so that complications like hypoglycemia, severe anemia or renal failure can be detected and treated promptly.

ASTHMA COMPLICATING PREGNANACY

Asthma is a condition where the hyperreactivity of the tracheobronchial tree leads to a temporary narrowing of the respiratory passages resulting in paroxysms of dyspnea, cough and wheezing.

Incidence

It affects about 5 per cent of the population. In a third of cases, it may improve during pregnancy; another third may show deterioration.

Etiology

The hyperreactivity of the respiratory tract to allergens, environmental pollutants or chemicals precipitate release of histamine, kinins and prostaglandins leading to narrowing, inflammation and secretions. This results in dyspnea, wheezing and cough till the lesion resolves or is reversed therapeutically.

Signs, symptoms and diagnosis

A pregnant mother with dyspnea and wheezing may give history of such complaints earlier. In a severe attack when the vital capacity is reduced to less than 50 per cent, the intercostal muscles are used for respiratory effort. Expiration is more difficult and prolonged; there is tachycardia and tachypnea. The diagnosis becomes obvious when the whole process gets completely reversed by using two puffs of a beta-adrenergic agonist.

Complications

The maternal hypoxia may lead to preterm labour, low birth weight and increased perinatal mortality. Status asthmaticus and pulmonary infections may occasionally present; these complications are difficult to manage.

Management

Management is the same as in the non-pregnant person. Asthma education in relation to pregnancy is useful. Treatment with oral salbutamol (4 mg) may be continued in a chronic condition. However in an acute attack she will need beta-adrenergic receptor agonist as inhalant 1–2 puffs every 20 min to a total cumulative dose of 5 mg/day. If there is no relief, hydrocortisone 2 mg/kg (or methyl prednisolone 40 mg) is given IV 6 hourly. In addition to oxygen, she is given ampicillin 2 g IV 8 hourly. Later, maintenance doses of beclomethazone as inhalant are adequate. Prostaglandin must never be used in any asthmatic. Asthma is no indication for induction of labour.

Bibliography

ACOG 2001. Gestational Diabetes. *Prac Bull* 30 (September)

Barbieri RC and Repke JT 2001. Renal disease in pregnancy. In: E Braunwald, AS Fauci et al (Eds) *Harrrison's Principles of Internal Medicine.* 15th edn. New York: McGraw Hill, 26-27.

Bondevik GT, Ulstein M, Lie RT et al 2000. Anemia in pregnant Nepali women. *Acta Obstet Gynecol Scand* 79: 341–49.

Branco M, Weiss, Ludwig V et al 1998. Outcome of cardiovascular surgery in pregnancy. *Am J Obstet Gynecol* 179: 1643–53.

Desai DK, Adanlawa M, Naidoo DP et al 2000. Mitral stenosis in pregnancy. *Br J Obstet Gynecol* 107: 953–58.

Expert Committee 2000. Diagnosis and classification of diabetes mellitus: a report. *Diab Care* 23(1): 54–519.

Guidotti R 2000. Anemia in pregnancy. *Br J Obstet Gynecol* 107: 437–38.

Gupta A, Lokhandwala Y, Saoshker P et al 1998. Balloon mitral valvotomy in pregnancy. *Am J Coll Surg* 187: 409–15.

Karnad AB and Rao KB 1994. Anemia in pregnancy: global view. In DR Popkins and LJ Peddle (Eds) *Women's Health Today.* London: Parthenon, 147–152.

Kochar DK and Thara R 2000. Cerebral malaria in pregnancy. *J Assoc Phys Ind* 47: 774–78.

Lapinsky SE 2001. Respiratory disease in pregnancy. *Curr Obstet Gynecol* 11: 153–59.

Nayak NC, Pande SK et al 1989. Etiology and outcome of viral hepatitis in pregnancy. *J Gastroenterol Hepatol* 4: 45–52.

Powers C 2001. Diabetes mellitus. In: E Braunwald, AS Fauci et al (Eds) *Harrison's Principles of Internal Medicine.* 15th edn. New York: McGraw Hill, 2109-42.

Ramachandran P 1999. Anemia in pregnancy. In SS Ratnam, KB Rao S Arulkumaran (Eds) *Obstetrics and Gynecology for Postgraduates*. Vol 1, 2nd edn. Chennai: Orient Longman, 46–55.

Rana Saad 2003. Heart disease in pregnancy. In SS Ratnam et al (Eds) *Obstetrics and Gynecology for Postgraduates* vol 2, 2nd edn. Chennai: Orient Longman.

Rao KB 1999. Jaundice in pregnancy. In: SS Ratnam, KB Rao and S Arulkumaran (Eds) *Obstetrics and Gynecology for Postgraduates*. Vol 1, 2nd edn. Madras: Orient Longman, 1–7.

Sadler L, McCown L, White H et al 2000. Pregnancy outcome with prosthetic valves. *Br J Obstet Gynecol* 107: 245–53.

Sawhney H, Suri V, Vasista K et al 1999 Pregnancy and congenital heart disease. *Austr NZ J Obstet Gynecol* 38: 266–269.

Sharma J and Gulati N 1991. Outcome of hepatic coma in pregnancy. *J Obstet Gynecol Ind* 40: 622–25.

Shaw K 1982. Cholestatic jaundice in pregnancy. *Am J Obstet Gynecol* 142: 621–25.

Stamm WS 2001. Urinary tract infections and pyelonephritis. In: E Braunwald, AS Fauci et al (Eds) *Harrison's Principles of Internal Medicine*. 15th edn. New York: McGraw Hill, 1620–26.

Tan JYL 2001. Cardiovascular disease in pregnancy. *Curr Opin Obstet Gynecol* 11: 137–145.

Wendel P 2001. Bronchial asthma complicating pregnancy. *Med Clin N Am* 28: 537–51.

White NJ and Breman JG 2001. Malaria. In: E Braunwald, AS Fauci et al (Eds) *Harrrison's Principles of Internal Medicine*. 15th edn. New York: McGraw Hill, 1203-1216

WHO 1992. *Prevalence of anemia in the world*. 2nd edn. Geneva: WHO.

WHO 2000a. *Expert Committee Report on Malaria*. Geneva: WHO, 44–45.

WHO 2000b. *Essential list of drugs*. Geneva: WHO, 25–26.

14. Neonatal emergencies

The newborn baby undergoes several physiological changes at birth. Occasionally, these changes do not occur in the way they should, making the newborn vulnerable to several emergency situations such as:

- Birth asphyxia
- Hypothermia
- Hypoglycemia
- Respiratory distress syndrome (RDS)
- Hyperbilirubinemia
- Infection

These neonatal problems are more prevalent in low birth weight (LBW) and preterm infants. In this chapter, these neonatal emergencies as well as the management of the LBW infant will be discussed.

BIRTH ASPHYXIA

Neonatal hypoxia is the leading cause of perinatal mortality and morbidity in developing countries and is responsible for cerebral palsy, convulsions and delayed milestones due to hypoxic ischemic encephalopathy. In the fetus, the main organ for gas exchange is the placenta. At birth, this function is taken over by the lungs, which are fluid filled organs during intrauterine life. With the first breath certain complex cardiopulmonary changes take place. Any antepartum or intrapartum event interfering with these changes may result in perinatal hypoxia.

Table 14.1: Causes of hypoxia in the antepartum and intrapartum period

Antepartum factors	*Intrapartum factors*
Maternal anemia	Prolonged labour
Hypertension in pregnancy	Uterine hypertonus
Diabetes mellitus	Malpresentation
Prolonged pregnancy	Prolapse of cord
Intrauterine growth restriction (IUGR)	Meconium stained liquor
Rh isoimmunisation	
Narcotics given within 4 hours of delivery	Fetal bradycardia
Bleeding in II or III trimester, and others	Placenta previa

Although the need for resuscitation of the newborn infant is often predictable, such circumstances may sometimes arise suddenly. Hence it is essential that the skills and knowledge of neonatal resuscitation be taught to everyone working in the labour ward.

NEONATAL RESUSCITATION

Neonatal resuscitation can be divided into four sequential steps:

Step 1 Warming, drying, suctioning and tactile stimulation
Step 2 Positive pressure ventilation (PPV) with bag and mask or endotracheal tube
Step 3 Chest compression
Step 4 Medication and fluids

Warming, drying, suctioning and tactile stimulation
The infant is delivered in a warm draught-free area and is kept under a radiant warmer. The wet linen is removed. Wrapping the infant in a prewarmed blanket or placing the dried infant skin to skin on the mother's chest or abdomen, helps in keeping the baby warm.

The airway is cleared after placing the head in a neutral

or slightly extended position. The mouth is first sucked followed by the nose, with bulb syringe or suction catheter (No. 8–10 F). Negative pressure of suction must not be more than 100 mmHg. Hence, regular suction apparatus is not to be used. Since aggressive pharyngeal suction can cause laryngeal spasm and vagal bradycardia, and delay onset of spontaneous breathing, deep suctioning must be initially avoided. Ideally, suctioning must be done after delivery of the head and before delivery of the shoulders except in 10 per cent of cases where the liquor is meconium stained.

Normally with suctioning most babies respond, cry, breathe well and remain pink with a heart rate of 100/min. In some babies, tactile stimulation like rubbing the back and flicking the feet may also be necessary.

Meconium aspiration may lead to atelectasis, chemical pneumonitis and edema. About 20 to 30 per cent of babies will have meconium in trachea; the vocal cords will then be meconium stained. In such cases the oropharynx and nasopharynx must be suctioned with a catheter followed later by endotracheal suctioning (using a laryngoscope). Drying and stimulation in such cases are done only after endotracheal suctioning.

Positive pressure ventilation (PPV) with bag and mask or endotracheal tube

The next important step in resuscitation is to give oxygen to the babies who are cyanosed, at the rate of 5–8 l/min through a face mask, or hand cupped around the oxygen tubing held 0.5 inch away from the nose till the baby turns pink. An infant who shows evidence of respiratory distress with cyanosis requires positive pressure ventilation using bag and mask at the rate of 40/min. Endotracheal intubation and suction is indicated in case of meconium aspiration, diaphragmatic hernia or when prolonged ventilation is required. The straight blade of the laryngoscope is used to view the larynx. After intubation, check the position by listening to breath sounds.

Chest compression

After about 30 seconds of bag and mask ventilation, evaluate the heart rate. If it is less than 60/min, chest compression should be initiated. Coordinate compression and ventilation and continue chest compressions till the heart rate is more than 60/min.

Medication and fluids

Medications are given via the endotracheal tube or the catheter into the umbilical vein. After 30 seconds of ventilation and chest compression if the heart rate is below 60/min:

1. Epinephrine is recommended IV or endotracheal (dose 0.1–0.3 ml/kg of 1:10,000 solution)
2. Volume expanders like normal saline or Ringer lactate 10 ml/kg is given as a slow IV push
3. Naloxone 0.1 ml/kg is specifically indicated if the mother has received narcotics. Bicarbonate is not routinely recommended. If scalp pH is low, a dose of 1–2 meq/kg or 0.5 meq/min, is given over 2 minutes intravenously, but only after adequate ventilation or perfusion is established (Wolkoff and Davis 1999; AAP/AHA 1994).

Special situations

1. Early elective intubation of extremely preterm infants (for example, < 28 weeks of gestation) may be necessary to establish airway. If necessary, a surfactant should be administered by the endotracheal route.
2. Multiple births require an extra person to immediately resuscitate the newborn. Apgar score is checked at 1 and 5 minutes to document post-resuscitation status.
3. If the baby has developed hypoxic encephalopathy, special intensive care will be required.
4. Discontinuation of resuscitation is recommended if spontaneous respiration and heart rate are not established even after 15 minutes of cardiorespiratory resuscitation.

HYPOTHERMIA IN THE NEWBORN

The normal axillary temperature of a newborn is 36.5–37.5°C. In hypothermia, it is below 36.5°C and in cold stress below 36.5–35.0°C. In moderate hypothermia it is 36.0–32.0°C and in severe hypothermia it is below 32.0°C.

Neonatal hypothermia continues to be an important cause of neonatal mortality. Newborns are vulnerable to extremes of ambient temperature as they do not have the capacity to produce enough heat for the surface area. Therefore there is a need to keep the baby warmer as compared to the adults. This situation worsens in preterm/ low birth weight, hypoxic or sick newborns. In addition, the baby loses heat by convection, evaporation and radiation.

Management

Preventive: 'Kangarooing' assists in the maintenance of temperature and facilitates bonding even in LBW babies. During transportation most babies develop hypothermia, so adequate measures are to be taken to provide warm transport in a transport incubator or along with the mother. Covering the head is essential since the heat loss from the head is more. Warm pink feet and body indicate that the baby is in thermal comfort. Hypothermia manifests as acrocyanosis, cool extremities, lethargy, bradycardia and apnea and leads to hypoglycemia, metabolic acidosis and hypoxia.

Curative: In cases of hypothermia rewarming should be done immediately, before cold injury sets in. In cold stress skin to skin contact, a warm room or bed and a 200 watt bulb radiant warmer will help. In moderate hypothermia the same measures will suffice, but it is essential to monitor the temperature every 15 minutes till normal temperature is reached. In severe hypothermia use of a radiant warmer and incubator are necessary till the temperature reaches 34°C. After this, slow rewarming is recommended. In addition, IV fluids like 10% dextrose solution and oxygen and supportive measures are also needed.

Complications

During rewarming, complications may occur. As rapid rewarming of the infant's body surface diverts blood from within, hypotension may occur. It has been suggested that the use of plasma expanders (normal saline or Ringer lactate) during rewarming improves survival. Abdominal distension is common and necrotising enterocolitis may also occur. Hemorrhagic pulmonary edema occurs if cold hypothermia persists. Mortality in severe hypothermia is 20–50 per cent.

HYPOGLYCEMIA IN THE NEWBORN

As glucose is essential for the brain and cardiac tissues to function, abnormally low levels of glucose may lead to encephalopathy; this has a potential for long term neonatal injury. Hypoglycemia is defined as plasma glucose level of less than 40 mg/dl in a term or premature infant. Dextrostix are only used for screening. However, plasma glucose levels should also be estimated to confirm the diagnosis of hypoglycemia. Clinical signs associated with hypoglycemia are tremors, irritability, jitteriness, hypotonia, tachypnea, pallor and feeding difficulties. It is commonly seen in infants of diabetic mothers, growth restricted babies, preterm, macrosomic babies and very sick babies with perinatal hypoxia, cold injury and sepsis. The best way to prevent it is by resuscitation, early breast-feeding and prevention of sepsis. The blood glucose levels of babies who are at risk should be checked periodically. Asymptomatic hypoglycemia should be treated if the blood glucose levels are below 25 mg/dl. Infusion of glucose 6 mg/kg/min is administered and glucose levels are rechecked after 60 minutes. The infusion should be continued till the baby reaches normal glycemia. It should not be given as a bolus to asymptomatic hypoglycemic infants. In symptomatic hypoglycemia a bolus of 2 ml/kg of 10% glucose solution at the rate of 1 ml/min is followed by a continuous infusion of glucose at a rate of 6–8 mg/kg/min and increased further to the rate required for maintaining normal glucose levels (40–50 mg/dl).

PERSISTENT SEVERE HYPOGLYCEMIA

If the baby needs more than 7.5 mg/kg/min of glucose, a pathological cause like congenital hypopituitarism, congenital adrenal hypoplasia and glycogen storage disease have to be ruled out. These conditions are rare and carry a poor prognosis.

HYALINE MEMBRANE DISEASE (HMD) OR RESPIRATORY DISTRESS SYNDROME (RDS)

About 30 per cent of all neonatal deaths result from RDS or its complications. It occurs primarily in premature infants. Other risk factors are maternal diabetes, genetic factors (RDS in siblings, male sex) and diaphragmatic hernia. The primary cause is inadequate pulmonary surfactant.

Clinical diagnosis of RDS is made when there is tachypnea, grunting, intercostal and subcostal retraction, nasal flaring, and cyanosis relatively unresponsive to oxygen. Breath sound may be normal or diminished with a harsh quality. Fine rales may be heard, mainly over the lung bases posteriorly. Chest x-ray in these cases show fine reticular granularity of parenchyma and air bronchograms.

Respiratory distress syndrome must be differentiated from pneumonia, cyanotic heart disease, diaphragmatic hernia, congenital anomalies of the lung and transient tachypnea of the newborn.

Prevention

The incidence of RDS can be brought down by antenatal administration of betamethasone or dexamethasone, 48 hours before delivery of the fetus if the gestation is less than 34 weeks.

Treatment

Apart from supportive care of LBW infants (which includes maintenance of temperature, calories and fluid balance), warm humidified oxygen should be provided at a base concentration sufficient to keep arterial level between 55 and 70 mmHg with stable vital signs. If the arterial oxygen tension cannot be maintained above 50 mmHg inspired oxygen concentration of 70%, applying CPAP at a pressure of 6–10 cmH_2O by nasal prongs is indicated. If an infant on CPAP cannot maintain arterial oxygen tension above 50 mmHg while breathing 100% oxygen or pH < 7.2, or has arterial blood PCO_2 of 60 mmHg or more or in case of persistent apnea, assisted ventilation is required.

Multidose endotracheal instillation of exogenous surfactant to LBW infants requiring 40% oxygen and mechanical ventilation for treatment of RDS has improved the survival rates in these neonates. Treatment with surfactant is usually initiated in the first 24 hours of life. Therapy is given via the endotracheal tube every 12 hours for a total of four doses. In premature babies if L/S (lecithin–spingomyelin) value of the liquor amnii done prenatally is less than 2, surfactant at a dose of 100 mg/kg may be given prophylactically in the first 5–30 minutes after stabilisation. It can also be administered to an infant born before 28 weeks within a few minutes of its birth. Additional complications due to RDS like metabolic acidosis, respiratory acidosis, complications of tracheal intubation and bronchopulmonary dysplasia have to be identified and managed.

NEONATAL SEIZURES OR CONVULSIONS

This is a common emergency in the neonatal period occurring in 0.1–0.2 per cent of term infants and 5–10 per cent of low birth weight infants. The immature babies are the most vulnerable because of the low level of the inhibitory neurotransmittors (GABA). Prompt diagnosis and immediate treatment will prevent neurological damage. Neonatal encephalopathy is a leading cause of convulsions occurring within 12–48 hours of delivery of an asphyxiated infant. The clinical manifestations vary in the neonatal period from subtle seizures, to tonic, clonic and myoclonic seizures. Subtle seizures are often missed since they include eye deviation, eyelid blinking, sucking, chewing, lip smacking and cycling movements with apneic episodes. Bradycardia may be the only manifestation in some preterm infants. Tonic convulsions occur in preterm and term infants and should be differentiated from decerebrate posturing. Multifocal clonic seizures are seen in term infants, especially hypoxic infants, and may be due to cerebral infarction. Myoclonic seizures are seen in CNS malformations and are severe in those with neurological damage; these have poor prognosis.

Apart from low perfusion encephalopathy other causes of seizures are intracranial hemorrhage, focal cerebral infarction, CNS infection (metabolic causes as in hypoglycemia, hypocalcemia, hyponatremia), congenital malformation of the brain and pyridoxine dependent seizures. In 40 per cent of patients, no cause may be detected. Benign familial seizures are characterised by clonic seizures occurring on the third day in term infants, due to mutation in chromosome 20. These seizures completely stop at the age of six months. Diagnosis is usually clinical, by good physical examination, keeping in mind the antenatal factors and the events cited above. Hypoglycemia and hypocalcemia should be considered in LBW babies and investigated. Blood counts, ESR, blood culture and cerebrospinal fluid examination may be necessary in cases of suspected infections. An EEG is done in the interval between seizures, especially in subtle seizures. If the EEG is normal, the prognosis is good and residual neurologic sequelae are less likely.

Management of seizures

Medications used to control seizures should be given

intravenously and there should be facilities available to ventilate the baby if necessary, as the majority of drugs also depress the respiratory centre. Phenobarbitone is still the drug of choice. A loading dose of 20 mg/kg is given. If fits are not controlled, an additional dose of 5 mg/kg can be given. (The maximum dose is 40 mg/kg). In case the seizures are not controlled, phenytoin 20 mg/kg IV, is given in two increments of 10 mg/kg each. If the seizures still persists, midazolam is given IV (200 μg/kg). Ventilation may be necessary when there is respiratory depression. For maintenance, give anticonvulsants (phenobarbitone 3–4 mg/kg/day orally). If phenytoin is also used it should be tapered to 3–4 mg/kg/day and stopped gradually. Phenobarbitone is continued for 6–8 weeks and stopped after a developmental assessment. If other metabolic disorders are diagnosed they are treated as in hypocalcemia and hypomagnesemia. Prognosis depends on the cause. Except in late onset hypocalcemia where there is normal development, in all the other causes there may be developmental delay.

NEONATAL SEPSIS

Neonatal sepsis is a clinical syndrome of systemic illness accompanied by bacteremia occurring in the first month of life. Incidence is about 0.1 per cent in live births. It is higher in infants weighing less than 1500 g. It may be of early or late onset and may be nosocomial.

EARLY ONSET DISEASE

This occurs in the first 5–7 days of life and has a multisystem manifestation with a fulminant course. The infant acquires the illness during the intrauterine period or peripartum due to ascending infection from the genital tract following chorioamnionitis. It may also acquire infection while passing through the birth canal during delivery.

Late onset disease

This is more common after the first week of life. Most of the organisms are from the postnatal environment, such as other babies or relatives.

Nosocomial infections

These occur more often in high-risk newborn babies such as low birth weight and premature babies, specially those in the NICU or in the incubator.

The early signs of infection include pallor, poor feeding, hypothermia, jaundice, apnea/tachypnea or chest retraction and tachycardia. It may develop mild ileus with associated abdominal distension or petechiae. Among the late signs of infection are cyanosis, grunting and respiratory distress, bulging fontanalles, convulsions, and DIC with bleeding from puncture sites.

Screening for neonatal sepsis includes WBC (total and differential) counts, C-reactive proteins, ESR, platelet counts, blood culture and culture of tissue fluids. Lumbar puncture and chest x-ray are done depending on signs and symptoms.

Treatment

Antibiotics should be given intravenously with careful attention to recommended dosage and frequency. Gentamycin (5 mg/kg) and ampicillin (50 mg/kg/dose) are the drugs of choice. In most cases where bacterial infection is confirmed by culture or where there is a strong clinical suspicion supported by a CRP rise, 7–10 days of appropriate antibiotic therapy is adequate. Immunoglobulin therapy has not yet proved to be beneficial. Exchange transfusion provides humoral factors and helps recovery from septicemia. Supportive therapy with IV fluids, warmth, feeding and maintaining nutrition are necessary for a good outcome. Neonatal tetanus can be prevented by giving tetanus toxoid to the pregnant mother. Perinatal viral infections occur due to toxmoplasmosis, CMV or HIV and these can be treated by giving appropriate medication during pregnancy to decrease vertical transmission to the infant.

NEONATAL HYPERBILIRUBINEMIA

Serum bilirubin in most infants rises to over 2 mg/dl in the first week of life. This reaches a peak of 6–8 mg/dl on the third day and falls by the tenth day. (The physiological range is upto 12 mg/dl.) In preterm babies it may go up to 15 mg/dl by the fifth day of life (physiologic hyperbilirubinemia). Hyperbilirubinemia has to be managed adequately if the physiological limits are exceeded. Bilirubin encephalopathy or kernicterus occurs when the toxic bilirubin damages the basal ganglia. The baby then develops lethargy, hypotonia and seizure. These may lead to death or long term disabilities. The goal of treatment is to prevent bilirubin concentration exceeding physiological levels. Phototherapy is the effective therapeutic approach. This changes the bilirubin through photoisomerisation into water-soluble bilirubin, which is excreted in urine. The maximum skin exposure (for example, double surface) helps faster excretion. Phototherapy is initiated when bilirubin levels are 12–15 mg/dl. If risk factors like prematurity, maternal isoimmunisation, sepsis, jaundice within 24 hours, perinatal hypoxia and other enzyme deficiency (G6PD) are present, early phototherapy may be initiated. Phototherapy may be stopped if the bilirubin levels decrease to less than 15 mg/dl.

Clinical management of hyperbilirubinemia in infants

If the bilirubin level justifies consideration of phototherapy, one should also investigate the cause of hyperbilirubinemia. This includes a clinically pertinent history of the mother, family history, type of labour and delivery, and infant's clinical course. Term infants who are clinically jaundiced at or within 24 hours of birth are not considered healthy and require

Table 14.2: Management of hyperbilirubinemia in a healthy term newborn

Age in hours	*TSB level in mg/dl (pmol/l)*			
	Consider phototherapy	Phototherapy required	Exchange transfusion, if intensive phototherapy fails	Exchange transfusion and intensive therapy
≤ 24	...	...	...	...
25–48	> 12 (210)	> 15 (260)	> 20 (340)	> 25 (430)
49–72	> 15 (260)	> 18 (310)	> 25 (430)	> 30 (510)
> 72	> 17 (290)	> 20 (340)	> 25 (430)	> 30 (510)

TSB: Total serum bilirubin
Phototherapy at these TSB levels is a clinical option. It may be used on the basis of individual clinical judgement.

further evaluation. Physical examination should be supplemented by laboratory investigations such as:

1. Serum total, conjugated and unconjugated bilirubin levels.
2. Blood group with direct antibody test (Coomb's test)
3. Hemoglobin and hematocrit values.

Optional tests (in specific clinical circumstances) include i) glucose-6-phosphate dehydrogenase (G6PD) screening; ii) serum electrolytes and albumin or protein concentrations. When bilirubin levels exceed 20 mg/dl or when dehydration is suspected.

Management is by phototherapy or exchange transfusion depending on the serum bilirubin levels as per Table 14.2.

CARE OF LOW BIRTH WEIGHT BABIES

The major cause of neonatal mortality is low birth weight. Low birth weight may be due to preterm birth or due to intrauterine growth restriction.

The following are the *standard definitions*:

Low birth weight	< 2500 grams
Very low birth weight (VLBW)	< 1500 grams

Extremely low birth weight (ELBW) < 1000 grams
Preterm birth: Gestational age at delivery is < 37 weeks
IUGR: Growth of the fetus is less than 10 per cent for the gestational age

About 10 per cent of all infants are born preterm or with IUGR. The majority of low birth weight babies are born in developing countries like India. The low birth weight here is due to maternal malnutrition, anemia, infection and poverty. Hard physical labour in the third trimester also slows down fetal growth. Preeclampsia, chronic hypertension, chronic renal disease and diabetes can cause LBW by decreasing blood supply to the fetus or because of preterm delivery. Prevention and management of spontaneous preterm labour by giving corticosteroids before delivery to prevent RDS, is a major step. This will reduce mortality and morbidity related to preterm and LBW baby.

The neonatal problems in LBW babies due to preterm delivery and IUGR are different. In the latter, the basic underlying mechanisms are growth restriction that has occured in utero and birth hypoxia. Due to lack of brown fat they are prone to hypothermia. Insufficient energy stores lead to hypoglycemia. They are prone to congenital malformations and intrauterine infections. The underlying morbidity in preterm babies are attributed to immaturity of organs, the most important being respiratory problems due to lung immaturity. Immaturity of the brain causes apnea, lack of co-ordinated sucking and swallowing, and hemorrhage including intraventricular hemorrhage. Immature metabolic pathway may lead to hypoglycemia, metabolic acidosis and hyperbilirubinemia. Insufficient humoral, cellular and mucosal immune mechanisms make them prone to infections. Excessive oxygen supplementation may cause blindness due to retinopathy of prematurity and bronchopulmonary dysplasia.

Delivery of low birth weight babies

Anticipatory guidance and preparation are necessary. At birth, the health professional who conducts the delivery should be experienced in resuscitation; a warm chain is essential. If such facilities are not available, in utero transfer to a tertiary centre is recommended.

Kangaroo care

1. Instead of using incubators, babies were nestled between the mother's breasts in an upright position when the mother and baby are discharged from hospital.
2. Instead of using formula milk, babies are fed breast milk, expressed by their mothers.

The advantages of this system are:

- Babies are kept warm by their mother's body heat.
- Nursing individually eliminates the risk of cross-infection.
- Feeding breast milk is a simple and inexpensive way of supplying nutrients; it is also fresh and free from bacteria.
- Mothers are actively involved in caring for their babies.
- Bonding between mother and baby is enhanced.
- Nursing also stimulates the mothers to produce more milk.

Feeding low birth weight babies

It is worth noting that the overall survival rate for the kangaroo project were high partly because it also included mature but small babies.

1. On the first day the fluid requirements range from 60 to 100 ml/kg (the difference between the three categories [LBW, VLBW and ELBW] being 20 ml/kg each).
2. The daily increment in all groups is around 15 ml/ kg till day 7.
3. About 20–30 ml/kg extra fluid should be added for infants nursed under a radiant warmer. For those receiving phototherapy an additional 10–15 ml/kg fluid should be provided.
4. These are general guidelines; the fluid therapy for each baby should be individualised.

For the first two days, intravenous fluids should consist of 10% dextrose only. After that sodium (2–4 meq/kg) and potassium (2–3 meq/kg) are also added to the dextrose. These requirements are generally met by preparing 1/5 isotonic saline (N/5) and adding 1 ml potassium chloride solution (15% in 100 ml infuscate).

For giving intravenous fluids to the neonate, a small volume infusion set (for electronic pump) should be used. The flow of fluids should be carefully monitored. Too rapid an infusion may result in congestive heart failure and even death in a small baby. Parenteral fluid therapy needs to be monitored carefully especially among babies weighing less than 1500 grams. Adequacy of fluid therapy is indicated by weight pattern in the expected range. A LBW baby loses 1–2 per cent weight every day amounting to 10–15 per cent cumulative weight loss during the first week of life. Birth weight is regained between days 10 and 14.

Vitamin supplements

All LBW babies should receive intramuscular Vitamin K 1.0 mg at birth. Vitamin A and D are required in doses of 100 IU and 400 IU daily, respectively, from age 14 days. Several of the available multivitamin preparations provide these doses in 0.3 ml (5 drops) volume. At 8 weeks of age, iron supplements should be started in a dose of 2 mg/kg/day. Very low birth weight babies (< 1500 g, < 32 week gestation) need vitamin E, calcium and phosphorus supplements till 37 weeks.

Prevention of infection

Low birth weight babies are predisposed to serious bacterial infections. The importance of preventing sepsis cannot be overemphasised. Hand washing by the health professional attending the delivery, by the mother and the family before handling the baby, and early and exclusive breast milk feeding are essential. Care of the umbilical stump and avoiding unnecessary interventions such as intravenous lines and needle pricks help in preventing infection.

Long term developmental outcome of LBW babies

India has higher rates of subnormal growth, health and developmental outcomes. The problems increase as the child's birth weight decreases. These handicaps include mental retardation, cerebral palsy, developmental delay, problems in cognition, attention and neuromotor functioning. The children must be followed up for 24 months. The majority of enrichment programmes have demonstrated improvements in developmental outcome.

Factors which affect long term developmental outcomes include social, environmental and biological factors. Poverty and illiteracy are the major factors.

The 'life cycle approach' for prevention of LBW pregnancies includes care of the adolescent girl, delaying pregnancy in young girls and providing education about parenting. Availability of comprehensive health care near her home reduces the risk of LBW.

According to Kramer (1987) specific public health interventions could reduce the prevalence of low birth weight in developing countries.

Interventions that could affect intrauterine growth are:

1. Dietary supplementation before pregnancy, during pregnancy or both
2. Reduction in the numbers of teenage pregnancies
3. Improvement in women's education
4. Reduction in work and energy expenditure during pregnancy
5. Efforts to reduce levels of smoking and tobacco chewing
6. Prevention and treatment of malaria

The first three interventions could also affect length of gestation.

Bibliography

American Academy of Paediatrics/American Heart Association 1994. *Textbook of Neonatal Resuscitation*. Dallas: American Heart Association.

Charpak N, Ruiz-Pelaez JG and de Calume Z 1996. Current knowledge of kangaroo mother invention. *Curr Opin Pediatr* 8: 108–12.

Dennery PA, Seidman DS and Stevenson DK 2001. Neonatal hyperbilirubinaemia. *N Engl J Med* 344: 581–590.

Kramer MS 1987. Determinants of low birth weight: methodological assessment and meta-analysis. *Bull WHO* 65: 663–737.

Manandar DS and Castelo A 2001. Diseases of the newborn. In JB Lawson, KA Harrison et al (Eds) *Maternity care in developing countries*. London: RCOG Press, 265–383.

Wolkoff LI and Davis JM 1999. Delivery room resuscitation of newborn. *Clin Perinatol* 26: 641–659.

15. Shock in obstetrics

Shock is a clinical syndrome resulting from inadequate tissue perfusion. In the absence of early detection and prompt intensive care it leads to multiorgan failure and death.

Incidence

Incidence is about 1 per cent of institutional deliveries.

Etiopathology

Depending on the causes it could be classified as:

1. Hypovolemic shock which is the most important cause of shock in obstetrics. It follows hemorrhages of pregnancy, mostly PPH, APH and ectopic gestation.
2. Septic shock is the next most common and follows unsafe abortions and puerperal infections. In this case the shock is due to bacterial toxins, endotoxins by Gram negative rods, exotoxins by the Clostridial group and enterotoxins by Gram positive bacteria.
3. Traumatic shock as in rupture of the uterus.
4. Neurogenic shock which follows inadvertent cephalad spread of spinal anesthesia.
5. Cardiogenic shock after an attack of AMI (acute myocardial infarction) in pregnancy.
6. Hypoadrenal shock that follows stress of an acute illness or major surgery in a case of adrenal insufficiency caused by chronic administration of exogenous glucocorticoids.

The hypoperfusion in shock leads to disparity between the supply and the need for oxygen and substrates causing cellular dysfunction, injury and release of inflammatory mediators further impairing perfusion in the microcirculation. The vascular tone is maintained by a balance between vasoconstrictors and vasodilators (Table 15.1). Initially, when the hypotension that accompanies shock causes a drop in the systolic BP to below 60 mmHg alpha-adrenergic receptors produce vasoconstriction to maintain blood flow to the vital organs (brain and heart) and to reduce blood supply to the other organs. Soon this hypoxia leads to a neuroendocrinal response, with secretion of some more vasopressors from the kidney (renin and angiotensins), adrenal (adrenaline, norepinephrine and aldosterone) and from the pituitary (vasopressin) to help increase the BP and the cardiac output. If however, the shock and hypotension worsen, the hypoxic cellular injury leads to production of inflammatory mediators, like TNF-α, nitric oxide, kinines etc. These vasodilators override the vasomotor tone causing intense and irreversible vasodilatation, worsening the hypoperfusion and end in death.

Table 15.1 Factors regulating the vasomotor tone

Vasoconstrictors	*Vasodilators*
Alpha-adrenergic receptors	Nitric oxide
Renin, angiotensins	TNF-α
Adrenaline, norepinephrine	Prostacycline, PGE_2
Aldosterone	Cytokines
Thrombaxane, PGF_{2a}	Lactic acid
Endothelin, vasopressin	K-ATP

Signs, symptoms and diagnosis

In the most common hypovolemic shock (of hemorrhagic origin), the clinical condition depends on the amount of blood/plasma lost. When the loss is mild (< 20 per cent of blood volume) there is mild tachycardia, slight sweating and anxiety. With moderate (20–40 per cent) loss, there is pallor, tachycardia (> 120/min), tachypnea (> 30/min), postural hypotension and oliguria (< 30 ml/min). When the hemorrhage exceeds 40 per cent, the classic picture of severe shock is seen. There is marked pallor and hypotension even in the supine position, with thready pulse and oliguria associated with agitation or mental confusion. The change from mild to severe shock may be slow or sometimes quite rapid in the elderly or in those with some other associated morbidity. In these cases of severe shock and hypotension, unless prompt and aggressive resuscitative measures are taken, it progresses to irreversible cell injury and death.

Shock can be diagnosed when there is hemodynamic instability, hypotension, pallor and the source of blood loss is obvious. In cases of plasma or fluid loss, diagnosis is more difficult. Acute blood loss is not associated with immediate changes in haematocrit, but in those with plasma loss, hemoconcentration is present.

In septic shock, during the early hyperdynamic phase, the extremities are warm, and the cardiac output increases but with no improvement in tissue perfusion. However, because the toxic agents, especially, lipopolysacharrides and nitric oxide continue to cause cell dysfunction, she develops ARDS, thrombocytopenia and DIC. With the onset of the hypodynamic phase, the cardiac output declines and limbs become cold; renal failure and death follows.

Prognosis

Prognosis depends on the cause and the interval between the onset of shock and intensive resuscitation. Chances of survival are best in hypovolemic shock following hemorrhage rather than in traumatic shock where there is tissue injury in addition to blood loss. Septic shock carries the worst prognosis as 20–30 per cent of those with severe sepsis and 40–50 per cent with septic shock die within 3–4 weeks.

Management

Preventive: Good perinatal care, prevention of anemia and careful monitoring during labour to avoid undue delay in second stage are important. Cesarean section is better than a difficult and traumatic vaginal delivery. The prophylactic use of oxytocics in the third stage and of antibiotics in elective cesarean section and potentially contaminated cases (chapter 18) contribute to reduction of shock.

Treatment

Immediately transfer the patient to an ICU. The foot end of the bed is raised and she is kept warm. If possible a pulmonary artery catheter (PAC) should be used to measure the hemodynamic profile. A Foley's catheter is used to record urine output.

For volume restitution 2–3 litres of normal saline or Ringer lactate solution are given intravenously through a large bore needle over 15–30 minutes; adequate compatible blood may be given in case of hemorrhagic shock.

Dopamine infusion is started in cases of severe hypotension to augment cardiac output without increasing heart rate

Respiration, is supported with oxygen administered through an endotracheal tube or by mask at the rate of 8 l/min.

Parenteral broad spectrum antibiotics are given to prevent infection. Monitoring of temperature, pulse, respiration, urine output and estimations of Na, K, Cl, acid-base, creatinine and blood for coagulopathy (in abruptio placentae or in cases of suspected infection) are essential till she is stable for 24 hours. Simultaneously, the cause for the shock has to be treated, for example, arresting blood/plasma loss, or by surgery in a case of ruptured uterus.

Case Report

A 32-year-old gravida 3, para 2, an unbooked case with uneventful medical/surgical/obstetric history was admitted with complaints of abdominal pain and vaginal bleeding for the past 1 hour in the ninth month of pregnancy. On examination, her general condition was satisfactory except for slight anemia. The uterus was 34 weeks' size with mild contractions and slight tenderness. The head was fixed at the pelvic brim but fetal heart sounds were absent. Slight vaginal bleeding was noted. Her BP was 120/80 mmHg, pulse 90/min, Hb 9 g%, blood group O+. Clotting time was 7 min to form a firm clot; USG confirmed no FH movements and the diagnosis was abruptio placentae.

Vaginal examination showed well-effaced 4 cm dilated cervix with a tense bag of membranes. Amniotomy allowed 200 ml of blood stained liquor to escape. Vertex was at station –2 and there was no bleeding. On catheterisation there was 120 ml of clear urine. Oxytocin infusion of 5 units in 500 ml of 5% dextrose saline was started and the blood bank alerted. There was good progress of labour as 75 minutes later a dead baby 2.4 kg was born. Ergometrine 0.2 mg was given IV. Placenta with 500 g of retroplacental clots was delivered followed by a gush of atonic hemorrhage. Oxytocin 20 units was added to the infusion and run at a fast rate. As the uterus was still lax carboprost 250 µg IM and bimanual compression of the uterus was done. As this was still ineffective, an additional 250 µg of carboprost was injected into the myometrium directly. The uterus contracted and was felt to be firm as the bimanual compression was continued. By now she had lost about 1500 ml of blood in addition to the retroplacental clots. As a result of massive PPH, she was pale, restless, BP 60/?, pulse was very fast and just palpable. In the meantime she was infused with a litre of saline IV and 500 ml of Ringer lactate was also continued. An urgent call to the blood bank was made to send four more units of O+ blood. The first unit received earlier was started through another IV line on the other arm. Fortunately, coagulopathy had not set in. The anesthetist started the CVP line, raised the foot end of the bed, started a regulated dopamine drip and gave her oxygen by mask at 8 l/min. Soon the pulse improved to 140/min, BP 90/?. With four more units of blood she was stable (BP 110/70, pulse 106/min and urine output 60 ml/h) but pale. On the advice of the anesthetist she was given the sixth unit of blood and transferred to the ICU for observation. No dextran was used in this case.

Comments: PPH is the commonest cause of hypovolemic shock in obstetrics. The risk of PPH increases in cases of APH, multiple pregnancy and emergency cesarean section. Massive blood loss (above 2000 ml) is an acute emergency. In such a case a team leader should take charge to coordinate prompt and aggressive resuscitative measures involving the obstetric, blood bank, anesthesia and the ICU departments. Frequent 'PPH drill' should be practised in the labour wards so that there is no delay or confusion likely to cause worsening of shock and an avoidable maternal death. Fortunately in this case, coagulopathy did not complicate the management.

The steps to be taken in cases of septic shock are:

1. Aggressive volume expansion with crystalloid solutions
2. Oxygenation preferably with mechanical ventilation
3. Combat hypotension with vasopressor like noradrenaline or hydrocortisone > 100 mg 6 hourly, in addition to dopamine infusion.
4. Antibiotics like cephalosporins and metronidazole IV (chapter 18) till culture reports are available
5. Surgical debridement or drainage depending on the source of infection (including replacement of old catheters, drains etc) may be life saving.
6. Antiendotoxins have been found useful.

In neurogenic shock following the spinal anesthesia the marked hypotension is due to the arteriolar and venodilatation resulting in decreased venous return to the heart. Treatment involves large volume of fluid replacement to restore normal hemodynamics and giving noradrenaline to increase vascular resistance.

In hypoadrenal shock, hydrocortisone 100 mg IV every 6 hours is needed, in addition to simultaneous fluid replacement.

Bibliography

Landry DW and Oliver JA 2001. The pathogenesis of vasodilatory shock. *N Engl J Med* 345: 588–95.

Munford RS 2001. Sepsis and shock. In: E Braunwald and AS Fauci et al (Eds) *Harrison's Principles of Internal Medicine.* 15th edn. New York: McGraw-Hill, 799–804.

William G and Dluhy 2001. Shock. In: E Braunwald and AS Fauci et al (Eds) *Harrison's Principles of Internal Medicine.* 15th edn. New York: McGraw-Hill, 222–28.

16. Acute abdominal pain in pregnancy

Acute abdominal pain in pregnancy may be either due to direct complications of the pregnancy itself or to conditions that superimpose on an ongoing pregnancy, some of which may be aggravated by the pregnancy itself. The site of the pain, its nature and associated symptoms and signs help to establish the diagnosis. Determining the diagnosis by meticulous history taking and physical examination is important because some conditions such as pyelonephritis, urinary calculi and red degeneration of the uterus require only conservative or expectant management while other conditions like ectopic pregnancy, rupture uterus or acute appendicitis, require immediate laparotomy which may be life-saving. A rapid evaluation of the vital signs of the patient on admission and corrective measures should be immediately instituted if patient is in impending shock or is hemodynamically unstable. When laparotomy is performed, a vertical midline or right paramedian incision is preferred not only to save time but also because pregnancy can cause intra-abdominal organs like the appendix and ovary to be at a different anatomical location than is usual.

Obstetric causes of pain

Some of these conditions have been described elsewhere in greater detail. The common obstetric conditions causing acute abdomen in pregnancy are:

1. *Abortions*: In the first trimester, threatened, inevitable, incomplete or septic abortions may be associated with cramping pain in the lower abdomen (usually associated with bleeding per vaginum which may be scanty in threatened abortion or severe with the passage of products of conception in inevitable and incomplete abortions). Abdominal pain with foul-smelling discharge, fever and a history of interference with the pregnancy earlier suggests septic abortions (chapter 2).
2. *Ectopic pregnancy*: Acute pain abdomen in the first trimester associated with bleeding per vaginum and hemodynamic instability disproportionate to the vaginal bleeding, point to a diagnosis of ectopic pregnancy. The uterus is of normal size or just bulky, the os is closed, there is a tender mass in the adnexa and severe pain on movement of the cervix. Ultrasonography and endoscopy are useful when the patient is stable and diagnosis is in doubt but not when patient is in hemorrhagic shock as the diagnosis is obvious and ultrasonography and laparoscopy will only delay the treatment (chapter 2).
3. *Impacted retroverted gravid uterus*: This occurs when a retroverted pregnant uterus gets incarcerated in the pelvis beneath the sacral promontory, usually between 13 and 16 weeks of pregnancy, causing acute retention of urine and pain in the abdomen. Retention of urine occurs because the bladder is displaced upwards and forwards due to the retroverted pregnant uterus filling the pelvis; as a result the urethra is stretched and compressed against the pubic symphysis. Occasionally, she may experience overflow incontinence secondary to the urinary retention; the full bladder in such cases may be mistaken for the gravid uterus or an ovarian tumour. Ultrasonography and clinical examination after catheterisation help in resolving the differential diagnosis.

   Management: Slow decompression of the distended bladder with a Foley's catheter and postural treatment for about 24 hours is usually all that is required to relieve the patient of her symptoms. The uterus usually escapes out of the pelvis. Only very rarely is manipulation of the uterus required, and in extremely rare cases laparotomy to divide adhesions binding down the uterus has been described.

4. *Preterm labour:* Abdominal pain before 37 completed weeks may often be due to premature uterine contractions and is usually accompanied by slight vaginal bleeding or 'show'. The presence of palpable and intermittent contractions of the uterus, vaginal discharge and progressive cervical dilatation and effacement over a course of two hours confirms the diagnosis.

   Management: As a premature baby is prone to higher perinatal mortality and morbidity, it is essential to ensure that optimum neonatal care facilities exist in the centre where the patient with premature labour is being treated. If this is not possible, in utero transfer prior to delivery is preferred. Tocolysis is given to delay or arrest labour for at least 48 hours till the effect of corticosteroids (given to improve fetal pulmonary maturity) has set in (chapter 9). If delivery is inevitable, maternal and fetal condition is monitored meticulously in labour, neonatal resuscitation facilities and personnel are kept ready and vacuum extraction of the premature fetal head is strictly avoided.

5. *Abruptio placentae:* Abdomen pain in the late second or third trimesters of pregnancy with or without bleeding per vaginum with a tonically contracted uterus and point tenderness suggests abruptio placentae. Maternal and fetal condition will vary according to the extent of placental separation and blood loss, which may be mild (in revealed) or severe (resulting in fetal death and maternal hypovolemic shock in concealed accidental hemorrhage).

   Management: This depends on the period of gestation, the severity of abruption and associated findings like severe preeclampsia or coagulation defects (chapter 9).

6. *Acute polyhydramnios:* When a patient presents in the late second or third trimester with sudden onset of abdominal pain, and abdominal overdistension due to a tense uterus with fluid thrill, the diagnosis may be acute polyhydramnios. The patient may have nausea, vomiting or orthopnea. Ultrasonography confirms the diagnosis and may reveal the cause (usually congenital anomaly like neural tube defects in the fetus or multiple pregnancy).

   Management: Decompression of the uterus of amniotic fluid offers immediate relief to the patient. Tapping is done at a dependent area preferably under ultrasound guidance and liquor is released slowly in order to prevent complications of rapid decompression like abruptio placentae and premature labour. If fluid reaccumulates rapidly, indomethacin is given orally to the mother in a dose of 500 mg 8 hourly.

7. *Rupture uterus:* This is usually seen after protracted labour or in patients with a previous uterine scar. The patient has severe abdominal pain that may subside in intensity after the rupture has occurred. There is marked lower abdominal tenderness with loss of uterine contour, easily palpable fetal parts, absent fetal heart sounds and maternal shock. Vaginal bleeding is usually present unless the fetal head blocks the cervix or the rupture is incomplete as in lateral tear into the broad ligament or dehiscence of previous caesarian scar covered by intact peritoneum.

   Management: Maternal condition is stabilised first by restoration of blood volume with normal saline or Ringer's lactate, after which laparotomy is performed. After delivery of the baby and placenta, the uterine edges are trimmed and sutured. In lateral tears with broad ligament hematomas, subtotal hysterectomy may be required (chapter 7).

8. *Puerperal sepsis/endometritis:* This is usually seen due to

infection of the placental site or retained products of conception. Lower abdominal pain in a recently delivered patient who also has fever and foul smelling discharge with or without bleeding, immediately suggests intrauterine sepsis or puerperal endometritis as the cause. In severe cases, the patient may be in endotoxic shock and may have tachycardia, and hypotension without fever. Lower abdominal tenderness is present on palpation of the uterus and signs of peritonitis may be seen.

Management: As infection is usually polymicrobial, parenteral administration of broad spectrum antibiotics, usually ampicillin, gentamycin and metronidazole are the mainstay of treatment. Any retained products are gently removed either digitally or by ovum forceps. A culture swab may be taken from the endometrial cavity and blood culture may be sent before starting treatment (Rao 1994). However, what is isolated may not be the only causative organism. Blood transfusion may be necessary, especially for the patient with endotoxic shock. If fever persists in spite of 2 to 3 days of antibiotic therapy, peritoneal or pelvic pus collection should be suspected and confirmed by ultrasonography. The abdominal collection may be drained by laparotomy. Culdocentesis is necessary in pelvic abscesses followed by colpotomy (Fig 16.1). Rarely, a necrotic and grossly infected uterus may require subtotal hysterectomy.

Gynecological causes of acute abdomen associated with pregnancy

1. *Torsion of ovarian tumour:* Previously existing ovarian tumours or an enlarged corpus luteal cyst may undergo torsion or (rarely) rupture, causing acute pain abdomen and associated vomiting. As the changing size of the uterus may act as a rotating force, this condition is usually seen in the first trimester and in early puerperium after the uterus is emptied. The unilateral nature of the pain

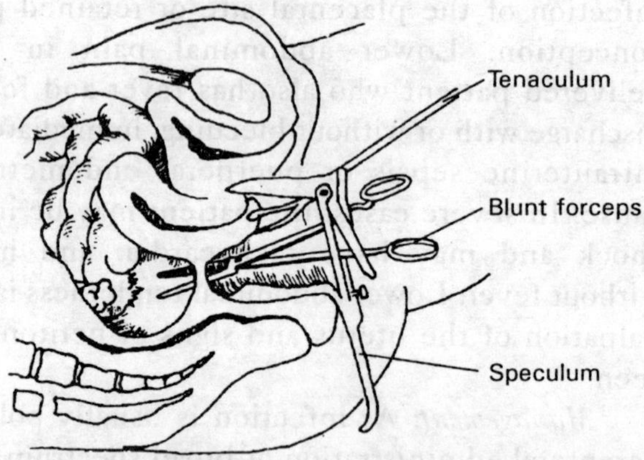

Fig 16.1 Colpotomy for pelvic abscess

(usually colicky) and a palpable, tense adnexal tumour suggest the diagnosis. Ultrasonography helps to establish the presence and probable nature of the tumour.

Management: In the first trimester if the pain abdomen is not severe, and only a partial torsion or drag of the ovarian ligaments is suspected, expectant treatment may be tried to avoid laparotomy and the hazards of general anesthesia in the embryogenesis phase. As the period of gestation increases, corpus luteal cysts may regress and simple cysts may be wedged against the enlarging uterus, and further torsion may be prevented only to recur sometimes soon after delivery. Solid tumours may be electively removed in the early second trimester. Severe abdominal pain, tachycardia and vomiting along with absence of ovarian flow on Doppler on ultrasonography suggests complete torsion of the ovarian pedicle and laparotomy and removal of the tumour is warranted at any stage of pregnancy in such cases.

2. *Red degeneration of uterine fibroids:* In this condition a patient presents with acute pain abdomen, nausea, vomiting, mild pyrexia and severe tenderness which is

located at one spot on the uterus where a fibroid may be palpated. When the physician knows about the prior existence of fibroids in the patient, diagnosis is easy; however, the absence of maternal hemodynamic instability and an otherwise relaxed uterus help to differentiate this condition from abruptio placentae. The diagnosis can be confirmed by ultrasonography.

Red degeneration occurs because the edema in the fibroid caused by the enlarging vascular uterus causes ischemia at its centre and resultant infarction. Management is purely expectant with rest, intravenous fluids in the acute phase, analgesics and prophylactic antibiotics.

3. *Hepatic rupture in severe preeclampsia:* This occurs in patients having severe preeclampsia and is often a progression of a hepatic subcapsular hematoma. The patient complains of severe epigastric or right hypochondrial pain, nausea and vomiting, and usually has other signs of impending eclampsia such as headache, high blood pressure and albuminuria. HELLP syndrome is usually associated and is often the cause of the hematoma. If the rupture is limited to the capsule, management is focused on the treatment of the preeclampsia. Rarely, if the capsule is breached the severe intra-peritoneal bleeding will require treatment of hypovolemia, analgesia and laparotomy for hemostasis.

Non-obstetric causes of acute abdomen

1. *Acute appendicitis:* This occurs in 1 of 1500 pregnancies. There is a greater incidence of morbidity and mortality when it occurs in pregnancy because of a delay in establishing the correct diagnosis and instituting early correction. As the uterus enlarges, it pushes the appendix upward and outward and the tenderness may be located high up in the abdomen and laterally in the flank, misleading you into making a diagnosis of pyelonephritis.

Also, the protective action of the omentum, which normally localises and limits infection, is inefficient as it is pushed above and over the fundus of the enlarging uterus. It is unable to reach the inflamed appendix, thus facilitating rupture and peritonitis. Fetal mortality can be as high as 30 per cent in patients with ruptured appendicitis. In advanced pregnancy, the inflamed appendix being distant from the abdominal wall, point tenderness may be absent and the patient complains of a generalised abdominal pain. Laparotomy in these cases is usually performed for a suspected diagnosis of abruptio placentae. A concomitant LSCS is not performed along with appendicectomy unless there is an associated maternal or fetal indication. In the case of a ruptured appendix, a drain has to be placed before closing the abdominal cavity.

2. *Urinary calculi:* Incidence is 1 in 1000–1500 pregnancies. Patients present with severe pain abdomen located usually at the flank or loin, radiating to the groin and often associated with vomiting and hematuria. Where there is a known history of renal calculi, diagnosis of the cause of pain is obvious, otherwise it is suggested by the nature and site of pain and the absence of uterine contractions with a relaxed uterus, ruling out labour as a cause. Microscopic examination of the urine may reveal presence of oxalate or calcium carbonate crystals and hematuria. Most calculi are visible on ultrasound. Radiological diagnosis of the calculus by x-ray or IVP may be deferred till after delivery unless the pain is intractable, persistent and fails to respond to medical therapy, and surgical intervention is contemplated. If IVP becomes necessary, a single film one hour after injection of contrast is sufficient for making a diagnosis.

   Management: Pain due to renal calculi can be relieved by parenteral analgesics and hydration in the acute phase. Small calculi (less than 0.5 cm) pass into the bladder in

50–70 per cent of cases because of the physiological hydroureter of pregnancy. Presence of pyelonephritis (which may set in secondary to the obstruction) may require antibiotic therapy. If medical management fails, surgical options are cystoscopic removal of lower ureteric calculi, ureteric stenting or even a ureterolithotomy. A percutaneous temporary nephrostomy may be required in very rare cases where there is protracted pain or sepsis, or persistent massive hydronephrosis with impaired renal function. Shock wave lithotripsy, being extremely hazardous to the fetus is contraindicated in pregnancy.

3. *Acute pyelonephritis:* This occurs in 1–2 per cent of pregnancies. The pregnant state predisposes to renal infection because of smooth muscle relaxation induced by progesterone; this leads to ureteric dilatation and stasis. This is further exaggerated in the right ureter because of the compression by dextrorotation of the growing uterus. Rarely, pyelonephritis may set in secondary to ureteric obstruction by calculi. The patient typically presents with acute pain abdomen (which may be colicky in nature and related to the affected flank), moderate to high grade pyrexia with chills and rigors, nausea and vomiting. There is severe tenderness and guarding in the affected renal angle and flank. Urine analysis reveals presence of pus cells, casts and epithelial debris. Urine culture and sensitivity will isolate the causative organism.

   Management is by adequate hydration by intravenous fluids, antipyretics, broad spectrum antibiotics parenterally till the culture results are obtained. Urine should be cultured periodically even if the patient is asymptomatic, as it is a recurring condition especially if the conditions predisposing to it (such as stasis in a dilated ureter secondary to uterine compression) persist.

4. *Acute cholecystitis:* The incidence of acute cholecystitis is reported to range from 0.5 to 0.8 cases per 1000 births.

This is almost always secondary to the presence of gallstones. It may be exacerbated by sluggish emptying of the gall bladder due to the effect of progesterone on its smooth muscle, leading to biliary stasis. The patient presents with unrelenting pain in the epigastrium or right hypochondriac area often radiating to the back, nausea, vomiting, mild to moderate grade pyrexia and occasionally mild jaundice. There is usually a history of previous attacks of spontaneously resolving colicky pain. While pregnancy seems to predispose to cholelithiasis, 50 per cent of these patients remain asymptomatic; symptoms are secondary to the onset of cholecystitis. The tenderness and rigidity in the lower border of the liver, a positive Murphy's sign and the presence of gallstones on ultrasound help to confirm the diagnosis. Management is conservative with intravenous fluids and parenteral antibiotics, nasogastric suction and analgesics. Very rarely, patients recalcitrant to conservative management may need surgery, that is cholecystectomy.

5. *Acute pancreatitis:* The incidence of pancreatitis is the same as in the non-pregnant state because pregnancy does not predispose to the condition and is found in about 1 in 3,333 pregnancies. Upto 70 per cent of these cases are associated with cholelithiasis; other causes are viral infections, hyperlipidemia and alcohol abuse. The patient presents with severe incapacitating epigastric pain, nausea, vomiting, abdominal tenderness and distension, and often low grade fever. Serum amylase levels are raised (over 1000 iu/l) as are serum lipase levels (over 5000 iu/l), which help to differentiate the condition from acute gastritis and acute cholecystitis with which it is often mistaken.

   Management is by intensive medical supportive care with intravenous hydration to maintain intravascular volume, withholding oral intake and analgesics. Nasogastric suction, proton pump inhibitors to inhibit gastric acid secretion and somatotropin analogues like octreotides are also given even though benefits have not been proven by randomized controlled trials. Electrolyte monitoring with replacement therapy is mandatory. Surgery is avoided, especially for the first 48 hours, and is resorted to only in cases with unrelenting disease and duodenal pseudocyst or peripancreatitic abscess formation.

6. *Intestinal obstruction:* Adhesions from the uterus to the bowel formed either as a result of previous severe pelvic inflammation or previous surgery may stretch, causing tenting or kinking of the bowel as the uterine pregnancy advances. This may cause intestinal obstruction and the patient then presents with acute colicky pain associated with nausea and vomiting and abdominal distension. Hyperperistalsis with exaggerated or 'tinkling' bowel sounds is a feature of small bowel obstruction. The pain tends to be constant and lower down in large bowel obstruction. Constipation is a symptom and the cecum may be palpably distended.

   Management: Conservative management with nasogastric tube and intravenous fluids may be attempted, but an obstruction severe enough to cause vomiting and abdominal distension and which does not respond to conservative management must be treated with laparotomy and division of the adhesions to prevent strangulation of the bowel.

Abdominal pain in pregnancy is therefore usually a manifestation of obstetric, gastrointestinal or genitourinary problems. Rarer causes are sickle cell crisis, pheochromocytoma, rupture of intra-abdominal vessel aneurysms and trauma causing hepatic or splenic rupture.

Although the majority of patients may report in pregnancy with pain abdomen due to minor problems like dyspepsia and gastritis, it may also be the earliest symptom of a potentially serious problem, making the diagnosis of the source vital. When the pain is not due to pregnancy complications, the diagnosis may be challenging due to the obscuring effect of the enlarged uterus. Conservative management based on relief of symptoms is the preferred option in pregnancy when diagnosis is not clear, unless deterioration of the general condition of the patient makes laparotomy necessary. Repeated examination at suitable intervals during which newer signs and symptoms will be elicited is the key to making the decision for surgery.

Bibliography

Baskett TF 2001. *Essential Management of Obstetric Emergencies*. 3rd edn. Chennai: Orient Longman.

Hope RA, Longmore JM et al 1998. The Acute Abdomen. In: *Oxford Handbook of Clinical Medicine*, 4th edn, 112–115.

Ramin KD and Ramsey PS 2001. Disease of the gall bladder and pancreas in pregnancy. *Obstet Gynecol Clin N Am* 28(3): 571– 80.

Rao KB 2003. Acute abdominal pain in pregnancy. In: SS Ratnam, KB Rao and S Arulkumaran (Eds) *Obstetrics and Gynecology for Postgraduates*. Vol 2, 2nd edn. Chennai: Orient Longman, 82–90.

Sawhney S, Gopalan S et al 1994. Urolithiasis in pregnancy. *J Obstet Gynecol Ind* 834–35.

Silen W 2001. Abdominal pain. In: E Braunwald, AS Fauci, et al (Eds) *Harrison's Principles of Internal Medicine*. 15th edn. New York: McGraw Hill.

WHO 2001. *Managing complications in pregnancy and childbirth*: abdominal pain in pregnancy. S 115–23.

17. Gynecologic emergencies

A gynecologist is often summoned to the emergency admission department to rule out a gynecological cause in a patient with abdominal pain. Where there are definite associated symptoms like bleeding or abnormal discharge per vaginum, a pelvic pathology may be obvious. However, gynecological problems may be present in spite of their apparent absence. For instance, a recently ruptured ectopic pregnancy may present with severe pain abdomen and signs of impending shock but bleeding may not yet have started. Twisted ovarian cysts or pedunculated fibroids may not be associated with bleeding.

An orderly and systematic history taking is vital after a rapid assessment of the general condition of the patient. A history of amenorrhea should alert one to the common causes of pain abdomen in pregnancy. It is important to rule out ectopic pregnancy and intraperitoneal bleeding as a cause of pain as it is one of the few conditions that is potentially life threatening and may require immediate laparotomy.

A gentle abdominal examination gives an indication of the likely presence of peritonitis, free fluid and masses in the abdomen. However, abdominal signs may be virtually absent in pelvic peritonitis, and careful pelvic and rectal examinations often reveal the diagnosis in patients with perforated appendix, diverticulitis, twisted ovarian cyst etc. Auscultation of the abdomen may reveal weak or absent bowel sounds which may indicate peritonitis.

Causes

Common causes of gynecological emergencies are described below.

1. *Acute pelvic inflammatory disease*: Infection of the uterine cavity, the fallopian tubes, ovaries and adjoining parametria gives rise to severe lower abdominal pain, often associated with fever and, occasionally, purulent, discharge per vaginum. This occurs most often due to ascent of sexually transmitted organisms and rarely secondary to gynecological procedures like D and C or IUCD insertion. The common causative organisms are Neisseria gonorrhoeae, Chlamydiae trachomatis, Mycoplasma hominis, Bacteroides, Escherichia coli, Peptostreptococcus and Gardnerella vaginalis. Infection in PID is often polymicrobial. Fever, vomiting and pain in the lower abdomen and pelvis are often preceded by symptoms of acute vaginitis and cervicitis (profuse purulent discharge and dysuria) as in neisseria and chlamydial infection. In 1 to 10 per cent of cases there may be perihepatic inflammation and adhesions (Fitz-Curtis syndrome). These patients will present with upper abdominal pain and hepatic tenderness that may be mistaken for acute cholecystitis. Clinically, there may be tenderness on palpation of the adnexae and uterus or evidence of masses in the adnexae in the event of pyosalpinx or tubo-ovarian matting indicating subacute or chronic infection. In severe PID with Gram negative infection, the patient may be in endotoxic shock. The absence of amenorrhea or a negative pregnancy test, presence of associated purulent discharge, leucocytosis and ultrasonography help to differentiate this condition from ectopic pregnancy. Swabs from the urethra and endocervix may help to determine the infective organism. Laparoscopy and laparotomy may occasionally be required for diagnosis.

   Management of PID is by antibiotics and anti-inflammatory agents where there is no obvious mass.

Masses that they persist in spite of antibiotic treatment may require surgical excision. As penicillinase producing and tetracycline resistant strains of N. gonorrhoeae are highly prevalent, treatment is preferably by single dose regimens like ceftriaxone 250 mg or cefotaxime 1 g intramuscularly or cefixime 400 mg or ciprofloxacin 500 mg orally. Where concurrent chlamydial infection is also suspected, azithromycin 1 g in a single dose orally or doxycycline 100 mg twice a day or erythromycin 500 mg four times a day may be given for a week. All sexual partners over the last two months should also be simultaneously treated.

2. *Rupture of corpus luteum:* Occasionally the corpus luteum may rupture with mild to moderate bleeding. Such patients will present with a history of severe pain abdomen and signs of intraperitoneal bleeding like tachycardia, pallor, mild abdominal distension and guarding which are often mistaken for a ruptured tubal pregnancy. The mid-cycle timing of the complaints, a negative gravindex test and presence of a hematoma in the ovary on ultrasonography point to the possible nature of the problem. As the condition is usually self-limiting supportive management normally suffices. A rare case of persistent or severe bleeding may require laparoscopy for aspiration of free blood and arrest of bleeding.
3. *Twisted ovarian tumour:* Torsion of an ovarian cyst may cause severe colicky pain in the lower abdomen, nausea and vomiting. On examination, the general condition is usually stable and a tender, tense mass may be palpable, separate from the uterus, anterior to it or in the fornices. Signs of peritonitis are usually absent unless there is a rupture of the cyst with irritation of the peritoneum due to the contents of the cyst, especially in dermoids. The pain may subside either spontaneously or with conservative treatment, only to recur later. Interruption of blood flow to the mass on Doppler ultrasound helps to confirm the diagnosis. Management is by laparotomy;

it should be performed early to prevent ischemic damage to the (remaining) viable ovary. If the ovary is infarcted due to chronic or repeated torsion of the pedicle with complete loss of blood supply, an ovariotomy may be required.

4. *Torsion of pedunculated fibroid:* An occasional pedunculated serosal fibroid may undergo torsion around its pedicle and give rise to severe abdominal pain. The general condition is usually good and there are no signs of peritoneal irritation. Severe point tenderness on palpation of the fibroid whether on abdominal or vaginal examination, suggests the diagnosis which may be confirmed by ultrasonography. Management is by abdominal or laparoscopic myomectomy or hysterectomy depending on the age of the patient and her parity.
5. *Ruptured endometriotic cyst:* Endometriotic cysts when large and tense can occasionally rupture, spilling its thick, tarry contents into the peritoneal cavity. The patient then presents with pain in the lower abdomen and signs of peritoneal irritation like mild abdominal distension, guarding and tenderness. Hemodynamic instability is usually rare. The remaining endometriotic cyst may be felt on vaginal or rectal examination. The uterus and adnexae may seem fixed and there may be severe tenderness in the posterior and affected fornices. Past history of menorrhagia with severe dysmenorrhea and pelvic pain and most often infertility, suggest the diagnosis. A negative pregnancy test and the presence of fluid with dense internal echoes help to differentiate this condition from ectopic pregnancy and PID.

   Management is by confirmation of the diagnosis by laparoscopy, when the cyst wall is removed and the abdominal cavity is washed well with normal saline to prevent formation of dense adhesions
6. *Ovarian hyperstimulation syndrome:* Patients undergoing ovulation induction with gonadotrophins (and sometimes

even with clomiphene citrate) may present with signs and symptoms resulting from high estrogen levels due to hyperstimulation of the ovaries. The patient has abdominal distension and pain, breathlessness and oliguria. Ascites and pleural effusion are seen; the symptoms depend on thc degree of ovarian stimulation and steroid production. Reduced renal perfusion, coagulation defects and electrolyte imbalance may be present due to intravascular space depletion and creation of 'third space' in the abdominal cavity. The presence of enlarged ovaries with multiple follicles and ascites on ultrasonography helps in the diagnosis.

Management is conservative with hospitalisation and bed rest. Vital signs are monitored and hematocrit, electrolyte balance, coagulation functions are regulated. Ascitic tapping may be required to prevent, and sometimes relieve, pulmonary symptoms. Surgery may rarely be required to correct torsion of the enlarged ovaries.

7. *Acute appendicitis:* Pain in the lower abdomen or right iliac fossa with nausea, vomiting and occasionally fever due to acute appendicitis is sometimes mistaken for gynecological conditions like PID or ectopic pregnancy. Tenderness is present higher up in the right iliac fossa with absence of bilateral adnexal tenderness as in PID. Absent adnexal mass, a negative pregnancy test and absent cervical excitation pain helps to rule out ectopic pregnancy as a cause of pain. Presence of fever, point rebound tenderness at the McBurney's point, leucocytosis on hematological examination and the visualisation of an edematous appendix with surrounding free fluid confirms the diagnosis. Treatment is by appendicectomy.
8. *Metropathia hemorrhagicum:* Occasionally, a case of juvenile metropathia is brought in with continuous menstrual bleeding. On examination, she may be

severely anemic. In such an emergency, compatible blood is transfused after grouping, typing and cross-matching to improve the general condition and steps are taken to arrest the bleeding by hormone therapy. Subsequent cycles will also need to be regularised after correcting the anemia. In a perimenopausal woman, profuse continuous bleeding may be due to carcinoma of the cervix or submucous myoma. A local examination including a speculum examination helps to confirm the diagnosis. In a case of cancer cervix, bleeding can be arrested by vaginal plug to ensure hemostasis and patient may need radiation after correcting the anemia. In a submucous myoma after correcting the anemia, surgical treatment is undertaken either by hysteroscopic myomectomy in a younger patient or hysterectomy. In these cases, endometrial carcinoma should be ruled out by curettage.

9. *Acute pyelonephritis and urinary calculi:* May cause severe pain in the lower abdomen with radiation from the flank or loin to the groin and a gynecological cause for the pain may be suspected. Presence of fever, absence of notable discomfort on palpation of the uterus and adnexa on vaginal palpation and an abnormal urinalysis result confirms the diagnosis. In case of pyelonephritis, urine culture helps to isolate the causative organism.

   Management is by intravenous hydration and appropriate antibiotic therapy.

Various other abdominal emergencies like a ruptured abdominal aneurysm, intestinal obstruction or volvulus, may be mistaken for gynecological emergencies if localising signs are found in the lower abdomen. A thorough and systematic history and examination helps to arrive at a diagnosis and management can be planned accordingly.

Bibliography

Arya OP 2001. Sexually transmitted diseases. In: JB Lawson, KA Harrison, S Bergstrom (Eds) *Maternity Care in Developing Countries*. Edinburgh: RCOG Press.

Hope RA, Longmore JM, McManus SK and Wood-Allum CA Year., *Oxford Handbook of Clinical Medicine*. 4th edn. Oxford: Oxford University Press.

Markas MD 1997. Pelvic Inflammatory Disease. In: JR Rock and JD Thompson (Eds) *TeLinde's Operative Gynecology*. 8th edn. USA: Lippincott-Raven.

Speroff L, Glass RH, Kase NG (Eds) *Clinical gynecologic endocrinology and infertility*, 6th Ed. London: Lippincott, Williams & Wilkins, 1115–20.

18. Antibiotics in obstetric and gynecologic emergencies

Antibiotics are used in obstetric and gynecologic emergencies mainly for the prevention and treatment of bacterial infections with a view to reduce morbidity and mortality both in the mother and her child. Sepsis or infections are responsible for 1 in 7 maternal deaths in developing countries. In gynecology, infections cause PID (with its sequelae), peritonitis, septicemia, endotoxic shock and death.

Principles

Antibiotics are classified depending on their mode of action (Table 18.1). Widespread and indiscriminate use of antibiotics has led to the development of resistant strains of bacteria. Therefore, care is taken when using them by following certain principles:

1. The bacteria should be susceptible to the chemotherapeutic agent.
2. The dose used should be bactericidal or at least bacteriostatic.
3. Combinations rather than a single agent is used for their synergistic action and also to prevent development of bacterial resistance.
4. Other factors to be considered are host immune status, associated pregnancy, toxicity, functional condition of the liver and kidneys and site of action (for example, brain, heart-valve vegetation, a closed cavity or bladder).

Table 18.1 Mechanism of action and bacterial spectrum of activity of groups of commonly used antibiotics

Group of commonly used antibiotic agents		*Mechanism of action*	*Bacterial spectrum action of activity*
i) β-lactam susceptible	Penicillin, ampicillin/ amoxicillin	Cell wall	Strep A and B; Clostridia; Spirochetes
ii) β-lactam resistant	Cephalosporins I-III generation	Cell wall	Gonococcus; Pneumococcus;
Macrolide	Erythromycin; azithromycin	Protein synthesis	Mycoplasma; pneumococcus; chlamydia
Tetracycline	Tetracycline; doxycycline	Protein synthesis	Chlamydia; granulomata
Aminoglycoside	Gentamycin	Protein synthesis	Urinary tract infections (UTI)
Sulpha	Trimetho- prim; sulfa- methoxazole	Cell metabolism	UTI; upper respiratory infections
Quinolones	Ciprofloxacin	DNA synthesis	UTI; gonococcus

5. When used empirically, it should be for a period of not more than 2–3 days, awaiting the culture report,
6. It should be clearly understood whether it is being prescribed for prophylaxis or for therapeutic purposes.

Prophylaxis

When an antibiotic is used as prophylaxis, the principles should be

- The likely severity of infection is greater than the side effects of the agent.
- It should be given for the shortest period needed to prevent target infections.
- It is given before the risk occurs (surgery) or soon after contact with infected individual.

It is advocated as a prophylaxis in the following conditions:

1. Cesarean section, both clean and high-risk cases,

cefoxitin or cefazolin is given soon after clamping the umbilical cord. Ampicillin 2 g may also be used as an alternative. Some advocate cloxacillin or a combination of ampicillin and clavulonic acid (beta–lactamase resistant) in such cases.

2. In abdominal or vaginal hysterectomy (clean and contaminated cases) similar antibiotics are given 30 minutes prior to and during surgery. In clean/contaminated/high risk genitourinary surgery ciprofloxacin 400 mg IM or IV before and during surgery is indicated
3. Prophylactic antibiotics are also used following vacuum aspiration and curettage in abortions and hydatidiform mole, PROM, prolonged labour, vaginal operative delivery, manual removal of placenta or any intrauterine manipulation. In all these cases ampicillin 500 mg six hourly may be given orally.
4. In infected or dirty cases as in ruptured uterus (handled outside the hospital), perforated appendix, ruptured tubo-ovarian masses or perforated uterus in unsafe abortions besides cefoxitin, metronidazole (7.5 mg/kg) is given IV six hourly against anerobic and Gram negative aerobic organisms before and for 3–5 days after the procedure. In these cases the antibiotics are used parenterally for the first 2–3 days and later orally, not only for preventive but also for therapeutic purposes as well.

In most cases however, based on the results of culture of the peritoneal fluid/pus and endometrial swabs obtained at the initial surgery, the antibiotics are changed if necessary. If the response is not satisfactory by the 4th or 5th day the patient should be thoroughly reviewed for any evidence of thrombophlebitis, pelvic abscess or adnexitis, and culture and sensitivity studies of blood and urine undertaken. Pus will have to be drained in cases of encysted peritonitis or in pelvic abscess. In infections with bacteroides the discharge has an offensive odour.

Table 18.2 Relative activity of commonly used antibiotics in PID

Antibiotic	*Chlamydia*	*N.gono*	*Vaginal anerobes Gram +*	*Vaginal anerobes Gram -*	*PID associated Gr rods*
Ampi/amoxicillin	++	++	++++	++	++
Doxycycline	++++	++	++	+	+
Cefoxitin	0	+++	++++	+++	+++
Cefotaxime	0	++++	+++	++	++++
Gentamycin	0	++	+	0	++++
Cipro	0	++++	+	0	+++
Mertronidazole	0	0	++++	++++	0

In obstetric cases the infections are usually polybacterial. The organisms most often involved are beta hemolytic streptococci, E.coli, Clostridia and bacteroides which are often found in the vagina or the anorectum. They become pathogenic when they find their way into the uterine cavity due to repeated vaginal examinations, especially after rupture of membranes, in the presence of trauma or hemorrhage. Care must be taken by the attendant nurse or physician to wear a mask, wash hands with soap and water repeatedly and reinforce the asepsis by the use of antiseptic cream and sterile instruments. This aspect of prophylaxis is as important as the use of antibiotics in the prevention and control of infections.

In polybacterial infections more than one antibiotic to which the organisms are susceptible should be chosen, such as, cephalosporins + metronidazole/gentamycin.

Table 18.3 Treatment of PID with combination of antibiotics for outpatients and inpatients

Outpatient therapy	*Inpatient therapy*
Ofloxacin 400 mg bid for 14 days	Cefoxitin 2 g IV 6 hourly
Plus	Doxycycline 100 mg IV or PO 12 hourly
Metronidazole 500 mg bid for 14 days	48 h after fever resolves, use outpatient regimen

In gynecologic conditions too the organisms are often polybacterial, though among STDs, Chlamydia trachomatis predominates. Even here it is often associated with N. gonorrhoeae, E. coli or other pathogens. In STD infections, the earlier the treatment of the infected individual and the sex partner, the less the tubal damage or severity of PID and its sequelae. Table 18.3 indicates the recommended lines of treatment in some of these infections.

Bibliography

Archer GL and Polk RE 2001. Approach to therapy for bacterial diseases. In: E Braunwald, AS Fauci et al (Eds) *Harrison's Principles of Internal Medicine.* 15th edn. New York: McGraw-Hill, 867–882

Holmes KK and Brunham RC 2001. Pelvic inflammatory disease. In: E Braunwald, AS Fauci et al (Eds) *Harrison's Principles of Internal Medicine.* 15th edn. New York: McGraw-Hill, 846–852.

Kasper DL 2001. Infections due to mixed anaerobic organisms. In: E Braunwald, AS Fauci et al (Eds) *Harrison's Principles of Internal Medicine.* 15th edn. New York: McGraw-Hill, 1011–17.

19. Analgesia and anesthesia in obstetric emergencies

Eternal vigilance is the price of safety.
Primum non nocere (First of all, do no harm)

The main aim of analgesia is to relieve pain in labour. This pain is of two kinds—visceral (i.e) due to ischemia, stretching and distensions of the lower segment and cervix through T10 to L1 mostly in the first stage and somatic (i.e) pain conveyed through S1 to S4 felt in addition in late first and second stages.

In spite of rapid advances in the art and science of obstetric anesthesia, these two age old dictums always stand as solid foundations for practice of anesthesia in obstetrics.

A woman in labour needing an anesthetic, poses multiple challenges to the anesthetist. Anesthesia related mortality accounts for 5 per cent of maternal deaths. An understanding of maternal physiology and pathology, a detailed history and proper examination of the patient coupled with necessary pre-operative investigations and assessment of the available facilities in a given institute (which vary considerably), will help the anesthetist to choose the best possible technique in a given situation.

Preoperative assessment

As is mandatory with any surgical patient, a proper and systematic preoperative assessment must be made in each case whenever possible, including for emergencies. A thorough clinical examination will help the anesthetist to select the most suitable anesthetic technique. A standardised set of investigations must be available like hemoglobin level, urine analysis, blood sugar level, blood urea, serum creatinine etc., for a proper assessment of the patient.

- It is always prudent to check the blood group and reserve enough blood in case of an emergency.
- In case the patient is anemic, transfusion of packed cells or whole blood should be given preoperatively.
- In a case of prolonged labour if there is dehydration and ketosis it has to be corrected prior to surgery.
- As far as possible, a thorough clinical history regarding previous surgery, or prior anesthetic complication, allergy to any particular drug and a complete history of present medication should be obtained.

A proper examination may reveal abnormalities involving the cardiovascular system (for example, valvular disease of the heart, hypertension), respiratory system (infections, bronchial asthma) etc. Of special importance to the anesthetist are the past history or presence of hypertension, diabetes, respiratory diseases, jaundice, use of steroids etc. In some parts of the world, certain groups or communities are known to have an abnormal metabolic response to certain anesthetic drugs (for example, prolonged apnea to suxamethonium). Many patients come out with relevant and useful information, provided a few leading questions are asked.

A special mention must be made about the examination of the airway. Individual variations like short neck, buck teeth, large breasts, large tongue, micrognathia, limited opening of the mouth, limited movement of the jaw should be noted. Ankylosing spondylitis, presence of a goitre, infections in the faciomaxillary area or epiglottitis, preeclampsia (resulting in laryngeal edema), or rarely tumours of the airway make intubation and maintenance of airway difficult.

Occasionally, in a pregnancy, airway edema may result

from hormone induced fluid retention, pregnancy induced hypertension (PIH) or excess weight gain. Repeated attempts to intubate may increase mucosal congestion, airway edema and cause bleeding. The anesthetist should consider the possibility of difficult intubation and problems of maintaining a proper airway, and should always be prepared with alternative techniques.

Mendelson's syndrome

It is of vital importance to consider the possibility of patients having had a full meal prior to admission for delivery on an emergency. Respiratory distress syndrome and pneumonitis from aspiration of gastric contents have been the most common cause of maternal deaths due to anesthesia in the past.

During pregnancy, there is delayed emptying of the gastric contents due to the effect of progesterone. Labour pain, fear, anxiety and the drugs used in labour may also contribute to delayed emptying of stomach contents. The gravid uterus also raises intragastric pressure, especially in supine and lithotomy positions. In subjects with hiatus hernia, the chances of regurgitation are greater. Sodium citrate 15 ml, 0.3 M preoperatively and H_2 blockers like ranitidine 50 mg IM are extremely useful for neutralising gastric acidity. Metoclopramide 10 mg helps in gastric emptying, increases esophageal sphincter tone and combats nausea.

In case of doubt it is essential to ensure that the stomach is empty. This is most commonly done through a nasogastric tube to aspirate the stomach contents. Other methods are with a gastric tube and by drugs like apomorphine 1–2 mg IV. Prevention of Mendelson's syndrome should be uppermost in the mind of the anesthetist dealing with emergencies.

In preventing aspiration of gastric contents, Sellick's maneuver is effective and life saving. Whenever intubation is attempted during cesarean section, an assistant is asked to push back the ring of the cricoid cartilage firmly and until the endotracheal tube is in place and the cuff is inflated, the firm pressure must be maintained without any relaxation.

The ideal anesthetic technique

The anesthetic must be one which provides

- Absolute safety (especially from problems like aspiration, hypotension, failed intubation and inability to maintain a proper airway)
- Absence of respiratory depression of the fetus
- Absence of awareness during surgery and psychological trauma to the mother
- Absence of toxicity to the mother and infant
- Rapid recovery as soon as the procedure is over.

One must always keep in mind the possibility of supine hypotensive syndrome of advanced pregnancy due to the gravid uterus pressing on the inferior vena cava (which drastically reduces venous return). Supine hypotensive syndrome can be prevented by placing a pillow under one buttock or by the lateral positioning of the patient.

GENERAL ANESTHESIA

Pre-medication

When cesarean section is decided upon, atropine 0.6 mg IM is given to prevent salivation and bradycardia. As a routine, no sedative or analgesic is administered, until the baby is delivered but the fact that pethidine might have been given during early labour must be kept in mind.

The standard induction technique is as follows: Pre-oxygenation for at least 3 minutes, thiopentone 4 mg/kg, suxamethonium 1.5 mg/kg, cricoid pressure, tracheal intubation and administration of nitrous oxide and oxygen, with a non-depolarising muscle relaxant. The non-depolarising muscle relaxant gallamine is not used in obstetric practice as it ***crosses the placental barrier and affects the fetus***. It is also never used in cases of renal impairment, as it is eliminated totally by the kidneys. Among the non-depolarising muscle relaxants, atracurium and vecuronium are useful because of their short duration of action, rapid clearance and minimal placental transfer. The risk of awareness can be avoided if a trace of volatile anesthetic agent is added (for example 1% isoflurane). Halothane is usually avoided because of its uterine relaxant property, but upto 0.5% is safe. Oxygen concentrations upto 66% are advocated, but there is always the fear of awareness during surgery. As all inhalation anesthetic agents cross the placenta, the interval between inductions and delivery should be minimised. As the need to maintain light anesthesia is only to prevent fetal respiratory depression, once the baby is delivered, the concentration of inhalation anesthetic can be increased or small doses of intravenous analgesics like morphine, pethidine, tramadol may be used.

General anesthesia is more risky than regional. Failed intubation occurs in 1 in 250 cases and is 10 times higher than in the non-pregnant.

Epidural block

Epidural analgesia is widely accepted as one of the most effective methods with an excellent risk-benefit ratio. The epidural space is a potential space that contains spinal nerve roots and the dural sac, areolar tissue, fat, lymphatics and the internal venous plexus, which becomes engorged during pregnancy, thereby reducing the volume of epidural space.

In this technique, as the woman is fully conscious, the anesthetist must obtain the maximum co-operation possible by being extremely patient and by explaining the procedure to her. Informed consent is taken. Continuous monitoring of pulse rate, blood pressure and fetal heart rate are mandatory. A drip is set up and pre-anesthetic hydration of the patient (for example, 500–1000 ml of Ringer lactate or 500 ml of colloid solution) is given. After putting the patient in lateral decubitus or sitting position, the epidural space is identified by the loss of resistance technique. Usually a 12G Tuohy needle is used after local infiltration at L2–L3 or L3–L4 lumbar interspaces.

The epidural catheter is inserted 3 cm into the epidural space. A test dose of either 3–5 ml of 2% xylocaine or 5 ml of 0.25% bupivacaine is injected into the epidural space and the patient is monitored for hypotension and paralysis. If there is none, a further dosage of 10–15 ml of analgesic solution (with 50 μg of fentanyl) is injected up the catheter to achieve a cephalad sensory T10 level of analgesia. After a few minutes, she is assessed for loss of sensation with a pinprick or dissecting forceps. If successful and the block is upto T10 level, the surgeon can proceed with the operation. The patient herself is the best judge as she will give information about the loss of sensation, heaviness and numbness of the legs or a feeling of pins and needles in the lower extremities apart from cessation of labour pains. It is important to monitor the blood pressure throughout as hypotension is a common complication. The catheter is kept in situ so that postoperative analgesia can be provided with an opioid analgesic like fentanyl, sufentanyl, alfentanyl, buprenorphine, tramadol etc.

Contraindications

The important contraindications for this method are untreated hypovolemia, refractory maternal hypotension, local sepsis, coagulopathy, maternal use of heparin within 12 hours of anesthesia, neurological diseases, maternal septicemia, patient's non-compliance and local technical problems due to anatomical deformities.

Complications

The two important complications are total spinal blockade and toxicity due to the injected drug.

1. Total spinal blockade: This serious problem must always be kept in the mind as the volume injected and the dose used, are both high. Usually it manifests itself as soon

as the epidural injection is given though it may even take 30 to 45 minutes for the full-blown picture to become apparent. The clinical picture can be frightening with marked hypotension, apnea, dilated pupils and loss of consciousness. Immediate management with ventilation, endotracheal intubation with 100% oxygen, elevation of legs and management of hypotension with fluids and vasopressors is required. If one is alert and prompt and resuscitative measures are taken, no unpleasant sequelae are likely.

2. Toxicity due to injected drug: It may occur either due to accidental intravascular injection or absorption from the extradural space. The patient will be disoriented, may have twitchings or convulsions and may even go into apnea. Management is by barbiturate or diazepam IV, intubation and intensive positive pressure ventilation. Protect the patient's tongue and teeth during convulsions.
3. Hypotension and cardiovascular depression: Management is by posture, oxygen, vasopressors, fluids and atropine in case of bradycardia.

Other complications include inadequate block, nausea and vomiting, epidural hematoma or abscess (rarely), dural puncture with subsequent severe headache.

Spinal or subarachnoid anesthesia

This is one of the simplest and most useful techniques in obstetric anesthesia which can be produced by performing a lumbar puncture at the level of L2–L3 or L3–L4 lumbar interspaces and injecting the local analgesic drug (5% xylocaine or 3 ml of 0.5% bupivacaine) directly into the cerebrospinal fluid. The anesthetic will act at the level of the lower end of the spinal cord and cauda equina. A nerve block to a level of T8–T10 will produce excellent anesthesia, suitable for a painless cesarean section.

Complications

The common complications of spinal anesthesia are:

1. The rapid onset of hypotension, which most often can be treated easily with IV fluids and use of vasopressor agents like ephedrine 5 mg. Pre-anesthetic hydration with either 500 ml of colloid or 1000 ml of Ringer lactate solution is advocated by many.
2. Post-spinal headache: It occurs in about 3 per cent of patients and is worse when the patient sits or stands and is often occipital in location. This can be prevented to a large extent by using a fine gauge needle (e.g. 25G) with a pencil point which separates rather than tears the fibres of the dura. Treatment is largely symptomatic with rest, analgesics, IV fluids, injection of normal saline 25–50 ml into the extradural space or injection of 10–20 ml of autologous blood into the extradural space to form a blood patch to seal the dural puncture etc., are some of the methods used to treat the headache.
3. Rarely there may be persistent backache, retention of urine, paralysis of the 6th cranial nerve causing diplopia and anterior spinal artery syndrome.

Caudal epidural block

Caudal analgesia is administered via the sacro-coccygeal membrane but is not preferred currently, due to difficulties in placement of a catheter, anatomical variations of the sacrum and requirement of high doses of analgesics.

Combined spinal-epidural technique

This technique combines the advantages of the spinal with the epidural analgesia, that is, rapid and effective analgesia for labour or cesarean delivery and postoperative pain relief. It combines a single subarachnoid injection for saddle block and the advantage of a catheter in the epidural space to raise the level of analgesia whenever necessary. The added advantage is that it gives immense satisfaction to the patient as she can walk, sit, void and bend down, all without pain.

Pudendal nerve block

This is the method of choice for simple forceps delivery. It produces analgesia of the perineum, the posterior two-thirds of the introitus and lower vagina. The transvaginal route is used to inject 1% xylocaine just behind the ischial spine. If the fetal head is too low, the transperineal route is used. If an episiotomy is to be performed, it is usual to infiltrate the line of the incision with a further 5 ml of 1% xylocaine.

Paracervical block

It can be of value in the first stage of labour, postpartum evacuation of the retained products or in cases of inevitable abortion.

Saddle block

Subarachnoid block with 5–10 mg hyperbaric bupivacaine given in the sitting position gives excellent analgesia for

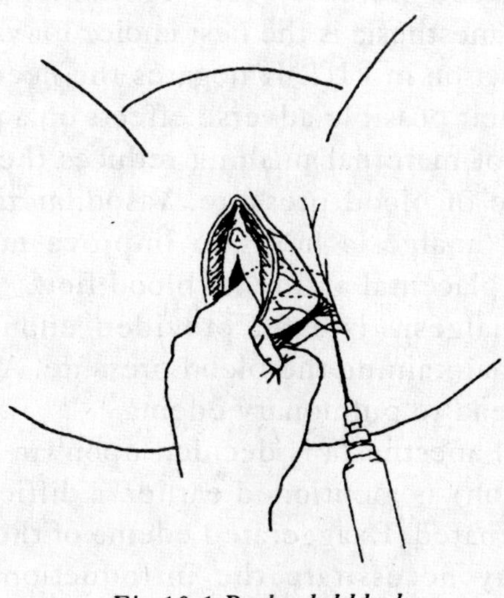

Fig 19.1 Pudendal block

stage II and instrumental vaginal delivery. For rapid onset of analgesia in late labour, stage I and stage II hyperbaric bupivaraine 5 mg is given with 25 micrograms fentanyl and 0.2 mg of morphine.

Subarachnoid narcotic analgesia

Drugs like morphine (0.2–0.5 mg), pethidine, fentanyl (25 μg), buprenorphine (0.1 mg), midazolam and tramadol are used to provide pain relief in labour when given intrathecally in small doses. The advantages are simplicity, safety and effectiveness with no motor or sympathetic blockade.

Undesirable side reactions are sometimes seen with morphine; there may be nausea, vomiting, retention of urine and pruritis.

ANESTHESIA FOR HIGH-RISK OBSTETRIC PATIENTS

Pregnancy induced hypertension

Magnesium sulphate is used for prevention and control of PIH. Hypotensives may also be used to control or to maintain the diastolic blood pressure below 110 mmHg.

Epidural anesthesia is the best choice for vaginal delivery or cesarean section in PIH. It negates the need for maternal opioids and their possible adverse effects on a preterm fetus. The absence of maternal pushing reduces the likelihood of associated rise of blood pressure. Vasodilatation associated with epidural analgesia helps to improve maternal blood pressure, and placental and renal blood flow.

Spinal analgesia is safe, provided enough caution is exercised in maintaining the blood pressure. Aggressive preloading may lead to pulmonary edema.

If general anesthesia is decided upon (in an emergency cesarean section) as mentioned earlier, a difficult intubation must be anticipated. Exaggerated edema of the upper airway structures may necessitate the introduction of a smaller endotracheal tube. Magnesium therapy potentiates all muscle relaxants, suxamethonium and atracurium being the least affected and vecuronium the most. Drugs like halothane, which sensitise the myocardium to catecholamines and drugs like ketamine and ergometrine, are contraindicated as they may elevate the blood pressure further.

Removal of the cuffed tube from the trachea at the conclusion of surgery should be considered only after return of the airway reflexes. It is always prudent to keep the patient in the intensive care unit for a day or two for proper and careful monitoring.

Hemorrhage

Obstetric hemorrhage is the leading cause of maternal mortality. Placenta previa, abruptio placentae, postpartum hemorrhage and ruptured tubal pregnancy are among the common causes of hemorrhage. In rupture of the uterus, trauma as well as hemorrhage leads to hypotension.

Preoperative assessment and grouping, awareness and early recognition, monitoring the blood loss during surgery/ delivery and prompt resuscitation go a long way in preventing an avoidable catastrophe. A good IV line, use of oxytocics and availability of blood are the most important factors in the treatment. General anesthesia is the technique of choice with minimal doses of cardio-stable drugs like ketamine, suxamethonium, atracurium, isoflurane etc. Resuscitation and anesthesia should proceed hand in hand. Ketamine is a useful drug for induction of anesthesia because of its cardio-stable effect and possibly its effect of increasing the uterine tone. This is usually followed by maintenance of anesthesia with 50% nitrogen oxide and oxygen combination and suxamethonium.

Complicated Vaginal Delivery

It is often difficult to decide the type of anesthesia to be adopted for a difficult breech delivery, shoulder dystocia, head entrapment and sometimes retained placenta.

For uncomplicated forceps delivery, pudendal block is the method of choice. General anesthesia is needed for many of these cases, which includes safe induction, good analgesia coupled with spontaneous respiration. Safety should never be compromised in these instances and they must be treated with as much care as in major surgeries. Regional techniques (especially if the epidural catheter is in place already) can be made use of, provided hypotension is avoided, as general anesthesia may cause some amount of neonatal depression. At times general anesthesia may not be possible due to practical considerations. For instance, most of these cases are conducted in labour rooms which do not provide the anesthetist with ideal conditions or properly trained theatre staff.

Heart disease

Detection and evaluation of heart disease is crucial for planning management of anesthesia during labour and delivery. Mitral stenosis and mitral regurgitation are the commonest cardiac valvular defects seen in pregnancy. The aim of the anesthetist should be to minimise the dangerous hemodynamic changes and Valsalva maneuvers and allow assisted delivery without maternal effort. General or epidural anesthesia can be safely provided for cesarean section. If general anesthesia is selected, drugs that cause tachycardia and events that increase pulmonary vascular resistance like arterial hypoxemia and hypoventilation must be avoided.

Appropriate monitoring and careful fluid titration to maintain filling pressures and minimise afterload and tachycardia are of vital importance.

Conclusion

The safety of obstetric analgesia and anesthesia has improved during the last few decades due to the advent of safer drugs, techniques and better monitoring facilities. Monitoring patients with obstetric emergencies who are at risk, require the knowledge and skill of an experienced anesthetist who must be readily available. The thin line between life and death mainly depends on the experience and alertness of the person at the head end on many occasions.

Bibliography

ACOG Practice Bulletin No. 36 2002. *Obstet Gynecol* 100: 177–187.

Atkinson, Rushman and Davies (Eds) 1987. *Lee's Synopsis of Anesthesia*. 11th edn. Singapore: Butterworth-Heinemann, International Editions, 526–537, 690–736.

Cunningham, MacDonald and Gant (Eds) *William's Obstetrics*, 20th edn. Prentice-Hall, 379–397.

Ezri T, Szmuk P, Evron S et al 2001. Difficult airway in obstetrical anesthesia. *Obstet Gynecol Surv* 56(10): 631–41.

Harmer M 2000. Analgesia and anesthesia. In: G Chamberlain (Ed) *Turnbull's Obstetrics*, 2nd edn. Churchill Livingstone, 591– 608.

Rodrigo N 2003. Anesthesia and analgesia in obstetrics. In: SS Ratnam, KB Rao, S Arulkumaran (Eds) *Obstetrics and Gynecology for Postgraduates*, vol 2, 2nd edn. Chennai: Orient Longman.

Scott BD 2001. Anesthesia for obstetrics. In: J Lawson, KA Harrison et al (Eds) *Maternity care in developing countries*. London: RCOG Press, 215–230.

Stoelting RK and Dierdorf SF (Eds) *Anesthesia and Co-existing Disease*, 3rd edn, Churchill Livingstone, 539–578

20. Critical care in obstetrics

Most patients, including pregnant women, are admitted to the intensive care unit for monitoring and treatment of life-threatening or potentially life-threatening vital organ failure. The human body has several mechanisms to compensate for excess demands placed on organ systems during illness. However, during pregnancy a significant part of this physiological cardiovascular, respiratory, renal and metabolic reserve is already used to meet increased physiological demands placed by the pregnant uterus and the developing fetus. As a consequence, chronic disorders or new intercurrent illnesses could result in severe organ dysfunction in pregnant women. In addition, several disorders unique to pregnancy including preeclampsia, intrauterine fetal death, acute fatty liver of pregnancy and amniotic fluid embolism could, by themselves, produce potentially fatal organ failure requiring intensive care.

Pregnant women form less than 1 per cent of all ICU admissions in the United States, but account for up to 7 per cent of ICU admissions in India. Medical disorders like autoimmune rheumatic disorders, urinary sepsis, pneumonia, asthma and hematological diseases account for most admissions in developed countries. On the other hand, multiple organ failure resulting from obstetric disorders like puerperal sepsis, septic abortion and intrauterine fetal death are the predominant indications for admissions in India (Table 20.1). Although the obstetric disorders mentioned are equally common in developed countries, early detection and

Table 20.1 Pregnant women with disorders requiring admission to medical ICU, K E M Hospital, Mumbai (n = 301)

Obstetric disorders	*No. of patients*	*Mortality (%)*	*Medical disorders*	*No. of patients*	*Mortality (%)*
Preeclampsia-eclampsia	135	23	Cerebral malaria	23	17
Sepsis	25	20	Viral hepatitis with hepatic coma	15	47
Abruptio placentae	23	13	Rheumatic heart disease	6	17
Postpartum hemorrhage	18	22	Poisoning	6	50
Cerebral venous thrombosis	17	24	Pneumonia	6	67
Acute fatty liver of pregnancy	16	31	Idiopathic thrombocytopenic purpura	2	50
HELLP syndrome	13	23	Severe anemia	3	0
Amniotic fluid embolism	1	100	Tetanus	1	100
			Acute leukemia	1	100
			Meningitis	1	0
			Typhoid	1	100

timely delivery prevent major maternal morbidity. In India, nonavailability or underutilisation of expert antenatal facilities in rural areas may limit early detection and treatment of high-risk pregnancies. Poor neonatal outcome of planned preterm delivery is another reason; many mothers decide to continue a high-risk pregnancy rather than opt for elective delivery at an earlier date, when explained the likelihood of survival of the premature infant ignoring risk to the mother.

Organ system failure in pregnant patients

Organ failure may result from worsening of pre-existing medical diseases like valvular heart disease or development of a new illness like pneumonia for the first time during pregnancy. Many obstetric illnesses too may result in acute severe organ dysfunction (Table 20.2). Unlike medical disorders, most obstetric disorders produce multiple organ

Table 20.2 Obstetric disorders producing multiple organ failure

Obstetric disorders	*Cardio-vascular*	*Renal*	*Hepatic*	*Coagulation*	*Respiratory*	*CNS*
Pregnancy-induced hypertension	+	++	+	++	0	++
Amniotic fluid embolism	++	0	0	++	++	0
HELLP syndrome	0	+	++	++	0	0
Acute fatty liver of pregnancy	0	++	++	++	0	++
Abruptio placentae	++	+	0	++	0	0
Rupured ectopic pregnancy	++	+	0	0	0	0
Intrauterine fetal death	0	+	0	++	0	0
Puerperal sepsis/ Septic abortion	++	++	0	++	+	0
Postpartum hemorrhage	++	+	0	++	0	0

Note: 0 = not affected, + = affected sometimes, ++ = commonly affected

failure which are rapidly progressive and also recover equally dramatically with appropriate intensive care. As a result, patients with obstetric diseases have a much better outcome than age-matched non-pregnant women admitted to the ICU.

Central nervous system (CNS) dysfunction

CNS dysfunction may present as seizures and coma. Seizures are a sine qua non of eclampsia. Seizures may also occur in patients with intracerebral hemorrhage due to coagulopathy, severe hypertension and cerebral cortical venous thrombosis. Pregnant women are also predisposed to getting cerebral malaria, and coma and convulsions may be a presenting feature in these patients. Other causes of coma are drugs used in preeclampsia including diazepam, chlorpromazine or magnesium, and hypoglycemia and metabolic encephalopathy due to fulminant hepatic failure.

In addition to treatment of the cause of coma, supportive treatment includes care of the airway, management of fluid and electrolyte balance and care of the skin and eyes. In most patients with a depressed cough reflex and pooling of pharyngeal secretions, endotracheal intubation is essential to prevent aspiration and to allow suctioning of tracheal secretions. Raised intracranial pressure due to cerebral edema or intracranial hemorrhage, may cause transtentorial herniation of the temporal lobes producing brainstem compression. Measures that effectively reduce intracranial pressure include intravenous mannitol (100 ml of 20% mannitol infused over 5 minutes, repeated 4 to 8 hourly). Short spells of mechanical hyperventilation may resolve transient increases in intracranial pressure.

Supportive treatment of status epilepticus includes an intravenous bolus of 25 per cent dextrose, 10 ml of calcium gluconate slowly intravenously, and correction of severe metabolic acidosis and hyperthermia. Convulsions are terminated by intravenous diazepam (5–20 mg injected slowly) or lorazepam (0.1 mg/kg, slow intravenous over 5 minutes). As anticonvulsant levels of diazepam are maintained for only 20–30 minutes, seizures may recur after this period. Lorazepam is preferred over diazepam as its effect persists for 6–12 hours. Intravenous phenytoin (20 mg/kg loading dose) should be diluted in normal saline and infused over 30 minutes to prevent recurrence of seizures. The maintenance dose of 100 mg 8 hourly should be continued thereafter. Magnesium sulphate is an excellent anticonvulsant in cases of severe PIH. However, patients having convulsinons despite magnesium should receive phenytoin. Intravenous phenobarbital (20 mg/kg at a rate of 50–75 mg/min) is administered for seizures persisting after phenytoin therapy. Hypotension and respiratory depression are common side effects of phenobarbital and must be promptly treated. Refractory seizures are treated by midazolam infusion. After an initial intravenous bolus of 0.2 mg/kg, an infusion at 0.1 to 0.2 mg/kg/hour is continued for 12 to 24 hours. Patients receiving benzodiazepines in large doses usually require endotracheal intubation and mechanical ventilation.

Cardiovascular dysfunction

The maternal blood volume increases by about 2 litres during pregnancy. Arterial blood pressure is unchanged but there is an increase in cardiac output by 30 to 45 per cent, mild increase in left ventricular end-diastolic volume and a decrease in systemic vascular resistance. Maternal body posture has an important effect on cardiac output after 20 weeks of gestation. Pressure of the gravid uterus on the inferior vena cava in the supine posture may cause a 30 per cent decrease in cardiac output.

Systemic arterial hypertension of varying degrees is a hallmark of PIH. Hypertension may be severe enough in some patients to cause left ventricular failure, especially when there is acute rise in blood pressure. Shock may occur due to several mechanisms. Hypovolemic shock may occur due to ruptured ectopic pregnancy, hyperemesis gravidarum, placental abruption, placenta previa, ruptured uterus and postpartum hemorrhage (Table 20.3). Pre/existing valvular heart disease may decompensate and manifest for the first time during pregnancy. Increased blood volume and increased cardiac output predispose these patients to developing acute pulmonary edema.

Table 20.3 Common causes of cardiovascular dysfunction in pregnant patients admitted to the medical ICU of K E M Hospital, Mumbai

Obstetric disorders	*No. of patients*	*Medical disorders*	*No. of patients*
Disseminated intravascular coagulation	52	Rheumatic heart disease	6
Preeclampsia-eclampsia	11		
Antepartum hemorrhage	8		
Postpartum hemorrhage	8		
Sepsis (puerperal, post-abortal)	4		
Total patients	83		6

Blood pressure equal to or above 160/110 mmHg can result in complications like seizures and cerebrovascular accident in the pregnant mother and requires rapid control. However, rapid reduction of pressure to normal levels may compromise placental perfusion and produce fetal anoxia. Blood pressure may be reduced by sublingual administration of nifedepine capsules (5 or 10 mg) containing the drug in gel form. This safely and effectively controls blood pressure in a majority of patients. Other alternative drugs include intravenous labetalol (10 mg initially followed by 20 mg every 20 minutes till blood pressure is controlled or a maximum dose of 80 mg is reached) or hydrallazine (5–10 mg at 20 minute intervals till blood pressure is controlled or a maximum dose of 40 mg is reached). Hypertension refractory to these drugs is an indication for intravenous nitroglycerine (10–50 g/min) or sodium nitroprusside (2–8 g/min) given by infusion pump. Prolonged use of nitroglycerine produces methemoglobinemia and cyanide toxicity in the mother and fetus. A rare complication of severe hypertension in pregnancy is dissecting aneurysm of the aorta which presents as retrosternal and interscapular pain and occlusion of one or more of the branches of the aortic arch. A parenterally administered beta-blocker like esmolol or metoprolol is the antihypertensive of choice in these patients.

Shock in obstetric practice is commonly hypovolemic (hemorrhagic) due to antepartum and postpartum hemorrhage and ruptured ectopic pregnancy. Septic shock may occur in patients with occult chorioamnionitis following intrauterine fetal death, puerperal sepsis or septic abortion. Cardiogenic shock may rarely develop in patients with peripartum cardiomyopathy or valvular heart disease. After admission to the ICU, the first priority in patients with shock is to establish a central venous access by the percutaneous route for fluid administration and for monitoring cardiac preload. While central venous pressure (CVP) alone suffices in patients with hypovolemic shock, pulmonary artery wedge pressure (PAWP) is a better indicator of cardiac preload in septic and cardiogenic shock. Low CVP or PAWP suggest hypovolemia, and rapid infusion of intravenous fluids should be started. A normal CVP or PAWP may be present in many volume-depleted patients and a fluid challenge should be tried. Infuse 200 ml of normal saline or Ringer lactate over 5 minutes and reassess CVP or PAWP. If these increase by 5 mmHg (6 cm H_2O) or more, then repeat measurement after 10 minutes. If the CVP or PAWP increase by less than 5 mmHg or decrease after an initial rise, the fluid challenge is repeated till these values rise and stay elevated. At this stage, inotropic therapy should be started if hypotension persists. Dopamine is preferred in septic shock and dobutamine in cardiogenic shock. However, dobutamine may worsen hypotension by its peripheral vasodilator effect and is therefore not used unless mean arterial pressure is ≥ 60mmHg. Both drugs are given as an intravenous infusion through a central venous line (3–15 μg/kg/min). If hypotension persists despite dopamine infusion, noradrenaline may be tried, especially in septic shock in a dose of 0.01–0.07 μg/kg/min.

Pulmonary thromboembolic complications are extremely common in patients with primary pulmonary hypertension or left to right shunts (> 50 mmHg). Therapeutic anticoagulation should be considered in these patients throughout pregnancy.

During cardiopulmonary resuscitation in pregnant patients who suffer from a cardiac arrest, besides defibrillation, cardiac compression and other steps of CPR including drug therapy, the gravid uterus should manually be displaced to the right to relieve aortocaval compression. If resuscitation is not achieved in 5 minutes, emergency bedside cesarean section should be performed. Outcome data from the US shows that there is 70 per cent survival for infants delivered within 5 minutes of maternal cardiac arrest, which drops to 13 per cent if delivered after 6–10 minutes.

Renal dysfunction

Glomerular filtration rate increases by about 25 per cent by the fourth week of pregnancy and reaches 50 per cent above baseline levels by 16 weeks. The serum creatinine too, drops to 0.5–0.7 mg/dl and therefore creatinine values which are normal for non-pregnant women may actually signify mild renal insufficiency during pregnancy.

Azotemia may occur due to prerenal factors like dehydration and hypovolemia which result in renal hypoperfusion and decreased glomerular filtration. This needs to be distinguished from azotemia due to acute tubular necrosis, which may result if renal hypoperfusion is severe and there is prolonged or direct tubular damage by drugs (aminoglycosides), toxins (sepsis, poisoning), renal microvascular disorders (preeclampsia, disseminated intravascular coagulation) or hemoglobinuria (miscatched transfusions, severe malaria).

In prerenal azotemia, renal perfusion is decreased and the renal tubules absorb almost all the sodium and water in the glomerular filtrate. The urinary osmolality is therefore elevated (> 500 mOsmol/kg), with urinary sodium < 20 mmol/l, urine/plasma creatinine ratio > 40 and blood urea nitrogen (BUN)/serum creatinine ratio > 10. In contrast, when acute tubular necrosis has set in, the urine osmolality is < 350 mOsmol/kg, urinary sodium > 40 mmol/l, urine / plasma creatinine ratio is < 20 and BUN/serum creatinine ratio is 10. Rarely, azotemia may also be glomerular in origin and is diagnosed by demonstration of proteinuria in excess of 3.5 g / 1.73m^2 body surface area / 24 hours. Causes include preeclampsia and autoimmune disorders like systemic lupus erythematosus.

Management of acute renal failure requires insertion of a central venous catheter to monitor volume status. Most obstetric conditions which cause renal failure, including preeclampsia and antepartum and postpartum hemorrhage, are associated with hypovolemia (Table 20.4). Once adequate hydration has been achieved by infusion of crystalloids or colloids as indicated, 100 ml of mannitol, an osmotic diuretic, should be infused intravenously rapidly. Alternatively,

Table 20.4 Common causes of acute renal failure in pregnant patients admitted to the medical ICU of K E M Hospital, Mumbai

Obstetric disorders	*No. of patients*	*Medical disorders*	*No. of patients*
Preeclampsia-eclampsia	43	Cerebral malaria	9
Disseminated intrvascular coagulation	18	Viral hepatitis with hepatic failure	5
Sepsis (puerperal, post-abortal)	6	Tetanus	1
Antepartum hemorrhage	5		
Acute fatty liver of pregnancy	4		
Postpartum hemorrhage	1		
Total patients	77		15

40–100 mg of frusemide may be administered; the author prefers the former as it is less likely to aggravate hypovolemia. The next step in patients who remain oliguric is to infuse dopamine in a dose which produces renal vasodilatation (2 – 5 µg/kg/ml), in an attempt to prevent or delay the development of ischemic acute tubular necrosis. The role of dopamine in renal failure in sepsis has been extensively debated and is now believed to be of little use, but to date there are no studies in obstetric patients. Patients with established renal failure will not respond to the above measures and are treated by conservative methods. These include fluid restriction to 600 ml plus the 24 hours urine volume, restriction of dietary potassium intake, provision of 0.8 g/kg body weight of protein which is rich in essential amino acids, and correction of metabolic acidosis. Approximately 70 per cent of patients recover with conservative treatment while 30 per cent require dialysis. Indications for dialysis are – severe azotemia (creatinine > 9 mg/dl), refractory acidosis, severe hyperkalemia (serum potassium > 6 mmol/l), fluid overload with acute pulmonary edema and uremia (drowsiness, seizures). In patients with multiple organ failure or coagulopathy, slow continuous arterio-venous or veno-venous dialysis using high-flux biocompatible dialysers is preferred to conventional hemodialysis as it produces lesser activation of inflammatory mediators, resulting in better outcomes.

Another uncommon cause of acute renal failure unique to pregnancy is postpartum hemolytic uremic syndrome, characterised by progressive azotemia, microangiopathic hemolytic anemia and oliguria. The syndrome is suspected if no evident cause for renal failure is found and fragmented red blood cells (schistocytes) are seen on the peripheral blood smear. The cause of the hemolytic uremic syndrome is not known and prognosis is guarded as progression to chronic renal failure is common. Approximately 20 per cent of pregnant women with acute renal failure develop acute renal cortical necrosis, a condition which is rare in nonpregnant acute renal failure. Women with coexisting preeclampsia and DIC are particularly predisposed to this complication suggesting that ischemia due to hemodynamic and vascular factors is greatly potentiated by intravascular coagulation, producing severe renal ischemic damage. While patients with acute tubular necrosis have a complete recovery of renal function in 4 to 12 weeks, most women with acute cortical necrosis show little recovery, remain dialysis-dependent, and go on to develop chronic renal failure.

Coagulation disturbances

At full term pregnancy, there is a 150–250 per cent increase in levels of clotting factors in blood and a decrease in circulating levels of antithrombotic factors including Protein S and antithrombin III. Platelet counts too decrease marginally during pregnancy. Pregnancy has been considered to be a hypercoagulable state. The incidence of deep vein thrombosis and cerebral venous thrombosis is increased during pregnancy and the risk of thrombotic complications in the postpartum period is approximately twenty times higher than in the antepartum period.

Subclinical coagulation disturbances are common in preeclampsia, with isolated thrombocytopenia occurring in up to 18 per cent patients, HELLP developing in another 15 per cent and DIC occurring in 11 per cent. The HELLP syndrome is a complication of preeclampsia characterised by platelet activation with platelet deposition on intact endothelium, severe thrombocytopenia, microangiopathic hemolytic anemia, and elevated liver enzymes. Clinically significant coagulation disturbances may occur in 50 per cent of patients with eclampsia, amniotic fluid embolism and intrauterine fetal death if the dead fetus is retained for 5 weeks. Critically ill pregnant patients account for 41 per cent of all patients with DIC admitted to our ICU (Table 20.5).

DIC manifests primarily as postpartum hemorrhage. Other hemorrhagic manifestations include bleeding from venipuncture sites, hematuria, bleeding gums, upper gastrointestinal hemorrhage, and, rarely, intracranial hemorrhage. Bleeding from multiple sites is an indication for studying the coagulation profile including prothrombin time, activated partial thromboplastin time, fibrinogen levels, platelet count, fibrin split products and D-dimers. Elevation of fibrin split products to > 40 g/ml along with thrombocytopenia (platelet count < $100{,}000/mm^3$ and altered coagulation tests are characteristic of DIC. Patients with DIC may develop hemorrhage within the uterine myometrium and

Table 20.5: Common causes of disseminated intravascular coagulation in patients admitted to the medical ICU of K E M Hospital, Mumbai

Obstetric disorders	*No. of patients*	*Medical disorders*	*No. of patients*
Abruptio placentae	20	Cerebral malaria	3
Preeclampsia-eclampsia	19	Acute myeloid leukemia	1
Postpartum hemorrhage	8		
Acute fatty liver of pregnancy	7		
Sepsis (puerperal, post-abortal)	2		
Amniotic fluid embolism	1		
No cause found	11		
Total patients	68		4

uterine atony is common. The combination of coagulopathy and uterine atony produces profuse postpartum hemorrhage.

Treatment of DIC consists of replacement of lost red cells with packed cells, and correction of clotting factor and platelet deficiency by blood component therapy with the aim of maintaining the platelet count at 100,000 per mm^3 and serum fibrinogen level at 100 mg/dl. One unit of single-donor platelets will increase the platelet count by 5000 to 10000 per mm^3 and one unit of fresh frozen plasma will raise the fibrinogen level by 10 mg/dl. It should be realised that serum fibrinogen is easy to measure and hence is used as an indicator of clotting factor levels. However, replacing fibrinogen alone is not sufficient to correct the coagulopathy and fresh frozen plasma is the preferred blood component. Cryoprecipitate may be added if fresh frozen plasma alone does not raise serum fibrinogen adequately and also in patients with acute renal failure as it is more concentrated than fresh frozen plasma so smaller volumes may be used. Some authors recommend a bolus of heparin along with infusion of antithrombin III concentrates prior to initiation of blood component therapy. DIC reverses rapidly after delivery and prompt evacuation of the uterus is attempted under cover of blood component therapy.

Hepatic failure

Varying degrees of hepatic dysfunction and elevation of transaminases is seen in 24 per cent of patients with mild preeclampsia, 50 per cent with severe preeclampsia and 84 per cent with eclampsia. However, hepatic failure due to preeclampsia alone is unusual and prognosis depends on the extent of renal and cerebral affection. Intrahepatic cholestasis of pregnancy (IHCP) is common in the second and third trimesters of pregnancy, but has a benign maternal outcome. The potentially fatal liver diseases in pregnancy are acute fatty liver of pregnancy (AFLP), hemolysis, elevated liver enzymes, low platelets (HELLP) syndrome and acute viral hepatitis (Table 20.6).

Table 20.6 Common causes of hepatic failure in patients admitted to the medical ICU of K E M Hospital, Mumbai

Obstetric disorders	*No. of patients*	*Medical disorders*	*No. of patients*
Acute fatty liver of pregnancy	16	Cerebral malaria	3
Preeclampsia-eclampsia	10	Acute viral hepatitis	15
Postpartum hemorrhage	8		
Sepsis (puerperal, post-abortal)	6		
HELLP syndrome	4		
Amniotic fluid embolism	1		
Total patients	37		18

The exact cause of acute fatty liver of pregnancy is not clear. It is more common in preeclampsia, and nutritional factors, alterations in lipoprotein synthesis, and enzyme deficiencies in the urea cycle of mitochondria are some of the proposed etiologic factors. This disorder can rapidly progress to fulminant hepatic failure and hepatic coma if not detected early and pregnancy is not terminated early. The transaminases are elevated, but rarely above 500 iu/ml, serum uric acid is elevated and thrombocytopenia and coagulopathy are prominent. These features help differentiate this syndrome from viral hepatitis where liver enzyme elevation is greater, uric acid is normal or reduced and platelet counts are normal.

The HELLP syndrome is believed to be a part of the spectrum of the PIH syndrome, with vascular endothelial damage being the primary event. This leads to platelet consumption, microangiopathic hemolytic anemia and damage to multiple organs including the liver. There is anemia, reticulocytosis, indirect hyperbilirubinemia, elevation of serum lactate dehydrogenase levels and proteinuria. These features help to differentiate this disorder from viral hepatitis and AFLP. Maternal mortality may be up to 25 per cent from coagulation problems, renal, pulmonary and hepatic failure. This disorder too reverses rapidly after delivery.

Acute viral hepatitis B, C and E and rarely hepatitis A may progress to fulminant hepatic failure. However, the course of disease in pregnant women is no different from that in nonpregnant individuals except for hepatitis E infection. Incidence of viral hepatitis is 9 times more in pregnancy and maternal mortality may be as high as 20 per cent with hepatitis developing in the third trimester. Delivery should be attempted only after the coagulopathy and thrombocytopenia are adequately corrected by blood component therapy. Unlike with AFLP, HELLP syndrome and preeclampsia, evacuation of the uterus in viral hepatitis does not improve maternal condition.

Management of fulminant hepatic failure consists essentially of managing the complications of hepatocellular dysfunction. Very little can be done for the liver disease, except in AFLP and HELLP syndrome where prompt delivery results in rapid improvement in liver function. Maternal mortality can decrease from 85 per cent to 25 per cent with early recognition and delivery in AFLP. Cerebral edema with raised intracranial pressure is an important cause of death in fulminant hepatic failure. The patient must be placed at a 20° head high position, and intravenous mannitol (100 ml of 20% solution) should be infused over 5 minutes and repeated 4 to 8 hourly. In patients in whom intracranial pressure is monitored, short periods of mechanical hyperventilation are useful when the cerebral perfusion pressure (difference between mean arterial and intracranial pressures) falls below 50 mm Hg. Maintenance of fluid balance requires insertion of a central venous catheter and monitoring of central venous pressure. Hypotension is common due to absorption of toxic vasodilatory aminoacids and responds to hydration, dopamine and noradrenaline infusion. Renal failure may coexist in up to 40 per cent of patients and needs to be aggressively treated. Metabolic problems like metabolic acidosis, hyponatremia, hyperkalemia and hypoglycemia are associated.

A nasogastric tube should be placed and gastric contents intermittently aspirated to detect gastric hemorrhage. A diet rich in carbohydrate but with reduced protein content should be administered to limit ammonia production by intestinal bacteria. Neomycin (contraindicated in renal failure and before delivery), ampicillin or metronidazole should be administered enterally to eliminate ammonia-producing intestinal bacteria. Lactulose (30 ml, 3 to 4 hourly, till diarrhea occurs) is administered to maintain an acidic pH in the gut lumen and reduce absorption of ammonia. Parenteral alimentation may be necessary to meet the protein and energy needs. Coagulopathy and bleeding is managed with blood transfusion and blood component therapy.

Respiratory failure

There is an 18 per cent decrease in the functional residual capacity and 15 per cent reduction in the expiratory reserve volume of the lungs in pregnant women due to elevation of the diaphragm; the compromise of lung volumes is maximum in the supine position. On the other hand, tidal volume and respiratory rate increase, with 48 per cent increase in minute ventilation at full term. Airway function is unchanged.

Respiratory failure with hypoventilation (type II respiratory failure) may occur due to depression of the respiratory centre in the medulla oblongata in patients with status epilepticus, cerebral edema, cerebral hemorrhage or venous infarction, hepatic coma, and antiepileptic drugs including magnesium, chlorpromazine, opioids and benzodiazepines. These patients have increased pCO_2 in arterial blood and require tracheal intubation and mechanical ventilation till the underlying abnormality recovers.

More commonly, respiratory failure results from impaired alveolar gas exchange resulting in profound hypoxemia (type I respiratory failure). Medical disorders producing this include community-acquired pneumonia, severe asthma, pulmonary thromboembolism and miliary TB. Cardiogenic pulmonary edema may develop due to acute renal failure and severe hypertension. The acute respiratory distress syndrome (ARDS) may occur in amniotic fluid embolism, disseminated intravascular coagulation, acute fatty liver of pregnancy, aspiration of gastric contents (Mendelson's syndrome) and systemic sepsis (Table 20.7). This is characterised by damage to the alveolar-capillary membrane due to cytokines or toxins, resulting in exudation of intravascular fluid into the pulmonary interstitium and alveoli, producing ventilation perfusion imbalance and interfering with gas exchange. Damage to the pneumocytes which produce surfactant results in alveolar collapse and intrapulmonary shunting of blood.

Amniotic fluid embolism typically has a biphasic course with initial severe hemodynamic disturbances and hypoxemia. About 40 per cent of patients have disseminated intravascular coagulation and 70 per cent develop ARDS 12–24 hours later. Treatment is mainly supportive. Tocolytic-induced pulmonary edema is a rare cause of respiratory failure. It is believed to result from increased pulmonary capillary permeability, volume overload due to salt and water retention,

Table 20.7 Common causes of respiratory failure in patients admitted to the medical ICU of K E M Hospital, Mumbai

Obstetric disorders	*No. of patients*	*Medical disorders*	*No. of patients*
Preeclampsia-eclampsia*	28	Pneumonia	6
Disseminated intrvascular coagulation	13	Cerebral malaria	5
Shock	10	Rheumatic heart disease	4
Sepsis (puerperal, post-abortal)	6	Poisoning	3
Acute fatty liver of pregnancy	4	Tetanus	1
Amniotic fluid embolism	1		
Total patients	62		19

* Most patients had respiratory depression due to seizures, coma or anticonvulsant drugs

increased pulmonary capillary hydrostatic pressure, cardiac arrhythmias and myocardial ischemia.

Management of type I respiratory failure consists of oxygen supplementation by nasal prongs, which allow an inspired oxygen concentration of 24–32 per cent. Oxygen mask with or without a venturi device permits administration of up to 60 per cent oxygen. Non-rebreathing masks with a reservoir bag allow delivery of higher concentrations of oxygen. Patients whose arterial pO_2 remains below 60 mmHg in spite of these means of oxygen supplementation require tracheal intubation and high flow oxygen with a T-piece. If this is unsuccessful in improving oxygenation, mechanical ventilation is required. Mechanical ventilation is also indicated in patients with type II respiratory failure, shock, ARDS and patients with type I respiratory failure who develop respiratory muscle fatigue. Various strategies of mechanical ventilation including positive end expiratory pressure (PEEP) have been employed, with the objective of maintaining arterial $pO_2 > 60$ mm Hg. All modes aim at using the lowest mean airway pressure so as to cause minimal hemodynamic compromise and pulmonary barotrauma and volutrauma. Oxygen concentration should be below 60 per cent as higher concentrations can produce or worsen ARDS. Recent studies in ARDS have shown that modes with inverse inspiration to expiration ratio, low tidal volumes and prone ventilation may improve survival and shorten the duration of the disease.

Prognosis

Prognosis depends on early diagnosis of complications, and in many cases, rapid delivery of the fetus. Access to intensive care units too is important. For patients admitted to the intensive care unit, prognosis depends to a large extent on the number of organs that have been affected (Table 20.8). Prognosis seems to be worse in organ failure due to medical disorders (40 per cent) than due to obstetric disorders (28 per cent).

Table 20.8 Number of organs affected and outcomes in pregnant women admitted to the medical ICU of K E M Hospital, Mumbai (n=301)

No. of organs affected	No. of patients	Mortality (%)
0	4	0
1	75	5
2	78	10
3	78	44
4	40	60
5	20	70
6	6	100
Total patients	301	30.2

Conclusions

Pregnancy related disorders are an important cause of multiple organ failure in India. Failure to detect complications like preeclampsia, AFLP or DIC early is one reason for this. Even if detected early, continuation of the high-risk pregnancy till life-threatening complications occur, is another reason. While intensive care can help to reduce the morbidity and mortality resulting from these potentially fatal conditions, the emphasis should be on prevention, early detection and prompt delivery of the fetus, which alone can help decrease maternal mortality from these disorders.

Bibliography

Beique F and Ramsay JG 1997. Cardiopulmonary circulation in the critically ill. Garrard C, Foex P, Westaby S. Principles and practice of critical care. London: Blackwell Scientific, 3–32.

Bernstein D and Tripodi J 1998. Fulminant Hepatic Failure. *Crit Care Clin* 14: 181–197.

Bick RL 2000. Syndromes of disseminated intravascular coagulation in obstetrics, pregnancy and gynecology. *Hematol Oncol Clin North Am* 14.

Collop NA and Sahn SA 1993. Critical illness in pregnancy: An analysis of 20 patients admitted to a medical intensive care unit. *Chest* 103: 1548–1552.

Cotton DB, Janusz CA and Berman RF 1992. Anticonvulsant effects of magnesium sulfate on hippocampal seizures: Therapeutic implications in preeclampsia-eclampsia. *Am J Obstet Gynecol* 166: 1127–1136.

Dati F, Pelzer H, Wagner C 1998. Relevance of markers of hemostasis activation in obstetrics/gynecology and pediatrics. *Semin Thromb Hemost* 24: 443–448.

Eclampsia Trial Collaborative group. Which anticonvulsant for women with eclampsia? Evidence from the Collaborative eclampsia trial. *Lancet* 345: 1455–63.

Haddad B, Barton JR, Livingston JC et al 2000. HELLP (hemolysis, elevated liver enzymes, and low platelet count) syndrome versus severe preeclampsia: Onset at 128.0 weeks' gestation. *Am J Obstet Gynecol* 183: 1475–1579.

Karnad DR and Vasani J 1992. Dissemniated intravascular coagulation: a review with experience from an intensive care unit in India. *J Postgrad Med* 38: 186–193.

Locksmith GJ 1999. Amniotic fluid embolism. *Obstst Gynecol Clin* 26: 436–444.

Lowenstein DH and Allredge BK 1998. Status epilepticus. *N Engl J Med* 84: 970–976.

Mahutte NG, Murphy-Kaulbeck L, Le Q, Lolomon J et al 1999. Obstetric admissions to the intensive care unit. *Obstet Gynecol* 94: 263–266.

Marini JJ 1996. Evolving concepts in the ventilatory management of acute respiratory distress syndrome. *Clin Chest Med* l7: 555–575.

Mroz LA. Hypertensive disorders of pregnancy 1999. *Anest Clin North Am* 17: 679–691.

Nicolini U, Guameri D, Gianotti GA et al 1994. Maternal and fetal platelet activation in normal pregnancy. *Obstet Gynecol* 83: 65–69.

Parikh CR and Kamad DR 1999. Quality, cost, and outcome of intensive care in a public hospital in Bombay, India. *Crit Care Med* 27:1754–1759.

Pisani RJ and Rosenow EC 1989. Pulmonary edema associated with tocolytic therapy. *Ann Intern Med* 110: 714–718.

Ramin KD. The prevention and management of eclampsia, *Obstet Gynecol Clin* 26: 489–503.

Ramshesh P 1996. Critical care in pregnancy and pregnancy related disorders. Dissertation, M D (General medicine), Mumbai University.

Rizk NW, Kalassain KG, Gilligan T et al 1996. Obstetric complications in pulmonary and critical care medicine. *Chest* 110: 791–809.

Rufei UM. Safe motherhood. In: Striving for better health in South-east Asia. New Delhi WHO 2001: 79–81.

Sibai BM, Ramadan MK, Usta I et al 1993. Maternal morbidity and mortality in 442 pregnancies with hemolysis, elevated liver enzymes, and low platelets (HELLP syndrome). *Am J Obstet Gynecol* 169: 1000–1006.

Tobin MJ 2001. Advances in mechanical ventilation. *N Engl J Med.* 344: 1986–1996.

World Health Organization 1990. Severe and complicated malaria. *Trans Royal Soc Trop Med Hyg.* 84 (Suppi 2): 1–65

World Health Organization 1999. Health situation in the South-east Asia region 1994–1997. New Delhi: WHO Regional Office for South-east Asia, 51–55.

Worthley LIG 1994. Oxygen therapy. In: Synopsis of intensive care medicine. Edinburgh: Churchill Livingstone. 387–392.

List of essential drugs

This chapter gives a list of drugs essential for use in emergencies. They are listed according to their alphabetical order. In each drug the route of administration, dosage, and strength it is available is stated. The permission of the World Health Organization for including this information from their technical report no. 895 (2000) is gratefully acknowledged.

Anesthetics

General anesthetics

Ether	inhalation
Halothane	inhalation
Nitrous oxide	inhalation
Oxygen	inhalation
Ketamine	inj (HCl 50 mg in 10 ml vial)
Thiopental powder	sodium salt 0.5 g or 1 g as inj

Local anesthetics

Bupivacaine	inj (HCl 0.25%,0.5%[vials] for spinal 0.5% in 4 ml amp to be mixed with 7.5 % glucose solution.
Lidocaine	inj 1%, 2% (HCl) in vial inj 1%, 2% (HCl)+ epinephrine 1 in 200, 000 in vial inj for spinal anesthesia, 5% (HCl) in 2 ml amp to be mixed with 7.5% glucose solution.
Topical forms	2–4% (HCl)

Preoperative medication for short term procedure

Atropine	inj 1 mg [sulfate] in 1 ml amp
Diazepam	inj 5 mg /ml in 2 ml amp OR 5 mg tab
Morphine	inj 10 mg (sulfate or HCl) in 1 ml amp

NSAIDS, ANALGESICS, ANTIPYRETICS

Non-opioids

Acetylsalicylic acid	tabs 100–500 mg
Ibuprofen	tabs 200 mg; 400 mg
Paracetamol	tabs 100–500 mg; syrup 125 mg/5 ml

Opioids

Codeine phosphate	tab 30 mg
Morphine	inj HCl or sulfate 10 mg in 1 ml amp oral 10 mg tab
Pethidine	HCl inj 50 mg in 1 ml amp tab 50 mg; 100 mg

Other NSAIDs

Cetaminophen	tab 650 mg
Diclofenac	tabs 50 mg; 100 mg
Naprosyn	sodium tabs 220 mg; 550 mg.

ANTIALLERGICS AND DRUGS USED IN ANAPHYLAXIS

Chlorphenamine	tab hydrogen maleate 4 mg inj 10 mg in 1 ml amp
Dexamethasone	tab, 500 mg; 4 mg dexamethasone disodium phosphate inj 4 mg in 1 ml amp
Ephedrine (adrenaline)	inj 1 mg as HCl in 1 ml amp
Hydrocortisone	[as sodium succinate] 100 mg powder in vial for inj
Prednisolone	tab 5 mg

ANTIDOTES AND OTHER SUBSTANCES USED IN POISONINGS

Non-specific

Charcoal activated powder

Specific

Acetylcysteine	inj 200 mg/ml in 10 ml amp (as IV for paracetamol poisoning)
Calcium gluconate	100 g/ml in 10 ml amp [as IV for $MgSO_4$ poisoning]
Naloxone	inj 400 mg/ml in 1 ml
Sodium thiosulfate	inj 250 mg/ml in 50 ml amp
Sodium nitrite	inj 30 mg /ml in 10 ml amp
Methylene blue	inj 10 mg/ml in 10 ml amp

ANTICONVULSANTS AND ANTIEPILEPICS

Carbamazepine	scored tab 100 mg; 200 mg
Diazepam	inj 5 mg/ml in 2 ml amp [IV or rectal]
Magnesium sulfate	inj 500 mg/ml in 2 ml amp; 500 mg in 10 ml amp
Phenobarbital	tab 15–100 mg; elixir 15 mg/5 ml.
Phenytoin	capsule or tab 25 mg, 50 mg 100 mg [sodium salt]
Phenytoin	inj [sodium salt] 50 mg in 5 ml vial
Valproic acid	[sodium salt] enteric coated tab, 200 mg, 500 mg.
Clonazepam	scored tab 500 mg

ANTI-INFECTIVE DRUGS

Anthelmentics

1. Intestinal anthelmentics

Albendazole	chewable tab 400 mg
Mebendazole	chewable tab 100 mg, 500 mg
Praziquantel	tab 150 mg, 600 mg.
Pyrantel embonate	chewable tab 250 mg; oral suspension 50 mg/ml

2. Antifilarials

Diethylcarbamazine	tabs 50 mg, 100 mg [dihydrogen citrate]
Ivermectin	scored tab 3 mg, 6 mg.

3. Antischistasomal and other antinematode drugs

Praziquantel	tab 600 g
Triclabendazole	tab 250 mg

Antibacterials

1. β lactam group

Amoxicillin	capsule or tab 250 mg or 500 mg
Ampicillin	powder for inj 500 mg [sodium salt] in vial
Benzathine	benzyl penicillin 2.4 million iu in 5 ml vial
Benzyl	penicillin [sod or pot. salt] 1 million iu, 5 million iu in vial.
Cloxacillin,	capsule sodium 500 mg, 1 g; 500 mg/vial as inj
Phenoxymethyl	penicillin [pot. salt] tab 250 mg
Procaine penicillin	1g or 1million iu; 3 g [=3million iu]
Amoxicillin + clavulanic acid	tab, 500 mg+125 mg
Ceftazidime	[sodium]powder 250 mg /vial as inj
Ceftriaxone	sodium powder 250 mg /vial as inj

Other Antibacterials

Chloramphenicol	250 mg capsule; 1g as inj
Ciprofloxacin	HCl tab 250 mg
Doxycycline	HCl tab or capsule 100 mg
Erythromycin	stearate or ethyl succinate 250 mg tab / cap 500 mg /vial as powder for inj
Gentamycin	sulfate inj 10 mg, 40 mg/ml in 2 ml vial
Metronidazole	tab 200–500 mg; inj 500 mg in 100 ml vial, suppository 500 mg, 1 g.

Nalidixic acid	tab 250 mg, 500 mg
Nitrofurantoin	tab 100 mg.
Spctinomycin	HCl powder 2 g in vial as inj
Sulfadiazine	tab 500 mg
Sulfamethoxazole +Trimethoprim	tab 100 mg+20 mg; 400 mg+80 mg inj 80 mg+16 mg in 5 ml amp, 80 mg+16 mg in 10 ml amp
Trimethoprim	tab 100 mg, 200 mg
Clindamycin	capsule 150 mg, inj 150 mg as phosphate/ml
Vancomycin	HCl powder 250 mg in vial as inj

Antileprosy drugs

Clofazamine	capsule 50 mg, 100 mg
Dapsone	tab 25 mg, 50 mg, 100 mg
Rifampicin	capsule or tab 150 mg , 300 mg

Antituberculosis drugs

Ethambutol	HCl tab 100 mg; 400 mg.
Isoniazid	tab 100 mg; 300 mg
Isoniazid+Ethambutol	tab 150 mg+400 mg
Pyrazinamide	tab 400 mg
Rifampicin	capsule or tab 150 mg, 300 mg
Rifampicin+Isoniazid	tab 60+30 mg, 150+75 mg, 300+150 mg, 50+50 mg, 150+150 mg.
Rifampicin+INH +Pyrazinmide	tab 60+30+150 mg, 150+75+400 mg, 150+150+500 mg
Rifampicin+INH +Pyrazinamide +Ethambutol	tab 150 mg+75 mg+400 mg+275 mg
Streptomycin	sulfate powder 1g in vial as inj
Thioacetazone+INH	tab 50 mg+100 mg, 150 mg+300 mg.

Antifungal drugs

amphotericin	powder for inj 50 mg in vial.

Fluconazole	capsule 50 mg, inj 2 mg/ml in vial
Griseofulvin	capsule or tab 125 mg, 250 mg.
Nystatin	tab, 100,000 iu , lozenges and pessary 100,000 iu

Antiviral drugs

Antiherpes

Acyclovir	tab 200 mg, powder for inj 250 mg/vial

Antiretroviral drugs

Nevirapine	tab 200 mg, oral soln. 50 mg /5ml
Zidovudine	cap 100 mg, tab 250 mg inj 10 mg/ml in 20 ml vial oral solution 50 mg/5ml

Antiprotozoal drugs

Antiamebic and anigiardiasis drugs

Diloxanide	tabs 500 mg [furoate]
Metronidazole	tabs 200-500 mg; inj 500 mg in 100 ml vial

Antileishmaniasis drugs

Meglumine antimoniate	inj 30 % in 5 ml amp
Pentmidine	powder for inj 200 mg, 300 mg [isetionate] in vial.

Antimalarials

For curative treatment

Chloroquine	tab 100 mg, 150 mg [as phosphate or sulfate]; inj 40 mg/ml in 5 ml amp [as HCl, phosphate or sulfate],
Primaquine	tab 7.5 mg, 15 mg [as diphosphate]
Quinine	tab 300 mg [as bisulfate or sulfate]
Quinine	HCl inj 300 mg/ml in 2 ml amp
Mefloquine	HCl tab 250 mg to be used with quinine.
Sulfadoxin +Pyrimethamine	tab 500 mg+25 mg
Artemether	inj 80 mg /ml in 1ml amp

Artesenuate	tab 50 mg

For prophylaxis

Chloroquine	tab 150 mg
Mefloquine	tab 250 mg
Proguanil	100 mg along with chloroquine

Drugs affecting blood

Antianemia drugs

Ferrous salt	tab, equivalent to 60 mg iron
Ferrous salt+Folic acid [as nutritional supplementation pregnancy]	tab 60 mg iron+400 mg folic acid.
Hydrocobalamin	inj 1 mg in 1 ml amp
Iron dextran	inj, 50 mg iron/ml in 2 ml amp

Drugs affecting coagulation

Desmopressin acetate	inj 4 mg/ml in 1 ml amp
Heparin sodium	inj 1000 iu/ml, 5000, iu/ml 20000 iu/ml in 1 ml amp
Phytomenadione	inj 10 mg/ml in 5 ml amp
Protamine sulfate	inj 10 mg in 5 ml amp
Warfarin [sodium]	1mg, 2 mg, 5 mg tab

Blood products and plasma substitutes

Dextran 70	injectable soln 6 %
Polygeline	injectable soln 3.5%

Plasma fractions

Factor VIII concentrate	dried
Factor IX complex [coagulation factors II, VII, IX, X]	concentrate dried.

CARDIOVASCULAR DRUGS

Antianginal drugs

Atenolol	tab 50 mg, 100 mg.
Glyceryl trinitrate	tab [sublingual] 500 µg
Isosorbide dinitrate	tab [sublingual] 5 mg
Verapamil	HCl tab 40 mg, 80 mg

Antiarrhythmic drugs

Atenolol and verapamil	as stated above.
Verapamil	inj 2.5 mg/ml in 2 ml amp
Digoxin	tabs 62.5 mg, 250 mg, inj 250 mg/ml in 2 ml amp
Lidocaine	HCl inj 20 mg /ml in 5 ml amp
Isoprenaline	inj 20 mg/ml in amp
Quinidine sulfate	tab 200 mg

Antihypertensive drugs

Atenolol	tab 50 mg, 100 mg.
Captopril	tab 25 mg.
Hydralazine	HCl tab 25 mg, 50 mg; inj 20 mg in amp
Hydrochlorothiazide	scored tab 25 mg
Methyldopa	tab 250 mg.
Nifedipine sustained release	tab 10mg
Reserpine	tab 100 mg, 250 mg inj 1 mg in 1ml amp
Prazosin	tab 500 mg, 1 mg
Sodium nitroprusside for infusion	50 mg in amp

Drugs used in heart failure

Captopril	scored tab 25 mg
Digoxin	tab 62.5 mg, 250 mg; inj 250 µg/ml in 2 ml amp

Dopamine	HCl inj 40 mg /ml in 5 ml vial.
Hydrochlorothiazide	tab 25 mg, 50 mg.

Antithrombtic drugs

Acetyl salicylic acid	tab 100mg
Streptokinase	powder for inj 100 000 iu, 750 000 iu in vial.

DERMATOLOGICAL DRUGS

Antifungaldrugs

Benzoic acid +salicylic acid	ointment or cream 6% + 3%
Miconazole nitrate	cream 2%
Sodium thiosulfate	soln 15%
Selenium sulfide	2% detergent based suspension

Antipruritic drugs

Betamethazone	ointment 0.1% calamine lotion;
Hydrocortisone	1% cream.
Scabicide:	
Benzyl benzoate	25% lotion.

ANTISEPTICS

Chlorhexidine	digluconate 5% solution
Polyvidone iodine	10% solution

DIURETICS

Amiloride	HCl tab 5 mg
Furosemide	tab 40 mg, inj 20 mg/ amp
Spironolactone	tab 25 mg
Hydrochlorothiazide	tab 25, 50 mg

Antacids and other antiulcer drugs

Aluminium hydroxide	tab 500 mg
Cimetidine	tab 200 mg; inj 200 mg in 2 ml amp
magnesium hydroxide	oral suspension [550 mg mg oxide/ 10 ml]

Antiemetic

Metoclopramide	HCl tab 10 mg; inj 5 mg/ml in 2 ml amp
Promethazine	HCl tab 10, 25 mg; inj 25 mg/ml in 2 ml amp

Oral hydration used in diarrhea

Salts for glucose-electrolyte soln	powder 27.9 g/l
Sodium chloride	3.5 g/l
Trisodium citrate dihydrate	2.9 g
Potassium chloride	1.5 g
Glucose	20 g/l

Contraceptives

Hormonal

Ethinyl estradiol +Levonorgestrel	30 mg+150 mg; 50 mg+250 mg [pack of four–for emergency contraception]
Ethinyl estrdiol +Norethisterone	tab 35 mg+1.0 mg
Norgestrel	tab 0.75 mg [pack of two for emergency contraception]
Levonorgestrel	30 mg tab

Medroxyprogestrone	
Acetate depot	inj 150 mg in 1 ml vial
Norethistrone acetate	200 mg oily soln as inj

Intrauterine Devices: Copper Containing

Barrier methods-condom with or without spermicide [nonoxinol]

INSULIN AND OTHER ANTIDIABETIC AGENTS

Glibenclamide	tab 2.5 mg, 5 mg
Insulin	inj [soluble] 40 iu/ml in 10 ml vial; 100 iu /ml in 10 ml vial
Intermediate-acting	
Insulin inj	40 iu/ml in 10 mlvial; 100 iu/ml in 10 ml vial [as compound insulin zinc suspension or isophane insulin]
Metformin	HCl 500 mg tab

IMMUNOLOGICALS

Anti-D immunoglobulin	
[human]	inj 250 mg in single dose vial
Antitetanus immunoglobulin	
[human]	inj 500 iu in vial
Rabies	
immunoglobulin	inj 150 iu /ml in vial.

MUSCLE RELAXANTS AND CHOLINESTERASE INHIBITORS

Alcuronium	inj 5 mg /ml in 2 ml amp
Neostigmine bromide	tab 15 mg; inj 500 µg, 2.5 mg [metisulfate] in 1 ml amp
Pyridostigmine	inj 1 mg/ml as amp
Suxamethonium	
chloride	inj 50 mg/ml in 2 ml amp

OPHTHLAMOLOGICAL PREPARATIONS

Gentamycin sulfate	0.3% soln as eye drops,
Silver nitrate	soln eyedrops 1%
Tetracycline	HCl as eye ointment 1 %.

OXYTOCICS

Ergometrine hydrogen maleate	inj 200mg in 1 ml amp
Oxytocin	inj 10 iu in 1 ml amp

ANTIOXYTOCIC

Salbutamol sulfate	inj 50 mg/ml in 5 ml amp

ANTIASTHMATIC DRUGS

Aminophilline	inj 25 mg /ml in 10 ml amp
beclomethasone dipropionate	aerosol inhalation 50 mg; 250 mg/dose
Epinephrine	HCl 1 mg in 1 ml amp
Salbutamol	tab 2 mg, 4 mg; inhalation 100 μg/dose; inj 50 μg/ml in 5 ml amp;
Respirator soln	for use in nebulizer 5 mg/ml
Theophylline	tab 100 mg, 200 mg, 500 mg

PARENTERAL SOLUTIONS

Glucose	5%, 10% [isotonic]; 50% [hypertonic]
Glucose saline	4% glucose 0.18% sodium chloride.
Potassium chloride	11.2% soln in 20 amp
Sodium hydrogen carbonate	inj 1.4%, 8.4% soln in 10 ml amp

VITAMINS

Ascorbic acid	tab 50 mg
Nicotinamide	tab 50 mg
Ergocalciferol	capsule 1.25 mg [50 000 iu]
Pyridoxine	25 mg tab;
Retinol sugar coated	tab 5.5 mg [10 000 iu]
Riboflavin	tab 5 mg
Thiamine	tab 5 mg

Appendix 1. Management of a hypertensive emergency

Clinical care is necessary in most obstetric and gynecologic emergencies to reduce the maternal mortality and morbidity. This chapter will consider some of the following conditions:

1. Severe PIH/eclampsia
2. Medical complications like
   a. Severe anemia complicating pregnancy
   b. Severe cardiac illness in pregnancy
   c. Acute renal failure in pregnancy
3. Hypertensive crisis complicating pregnancy
4. DIC
5. Hypovolemic shock

Of these PIH, eclampsia, anemia and hypovolemic shock have already been considered in chapter 4.

A hypertensive emergency is defined as a condition where acute target organ damage due to the blood pressure exceeding 169 systole and 109 diastole is brought down rapidly. It differs from hypertensive urgency were the blood pressure is gradually reduced over a few hours. The incidence of this condition is 7 per cent.

Malignant hypertension is a condition where diastolic blood pressure is 130 mmHg. It constitutes a complication of malignant hypertension and usually occurs in the scenario of diastolic blood pressure in excess of 130 mmHg. It is characterised by the occurrence of severe hypertension with neurological symptoms and/or signs. There is a school of thought which believes that eclampsia represents a form of hypertensive encephalopathy while others maintain that this cannot be the case as all eclamptic patients do not exhibit severe hypertension. There appears to be a shift in thinking that both eclampsia and hypertensive encephalopathy are considered to be part of reversible posterior leucoencephalopathy syndrome (PLS) which is diagnosed clinico-radiogically. It is important to note that PLS has multifactorial causes, many of which are non-hypertensive in origin.

In pregnancy, diastolic blood pressure of 110 mmHg or systolic blood pressure of 170 mmHg or greater, is regarded as a hypertensive crisis. It has been found that young women may develop complications such as encephalopathy with a diastolic blood pressure of 120 mmHg. It is thus important to lower high blood pressure once it reaches 110 mmHg in the pregnant patient. However, one should be aware of the fact that blood pressures are often labile (especially in the severe preeclamptic/eclamptic patient); in addition, sensitivity to acute acting antihypertensive agents should be taken into account. Very high blood pressure values should therefore be reduced promptly but gradually, as marked hypotension may complicate an overzealous attempt at blood pressure control. The recommendation is that diastolic blood pressure should not be reduced by more than 30 mmHg and neither should the mean arterial pressure (MAP) be reduced by more than 25 per cent. It is important to administer the drugs in small doses intermittently or by utilisation of a controlled infusion method. One should avoid the simultaneous use of more than one acute antihypertensive agent as a compound effect may be elicited. Postural hypotension would have a similar result; therefore, patients should be nursed on their sides or tilted with the aid of a pelvic wedge.

Management

The management of acute severe hypertension with target organ damage or hypertensive encephalopathy usually constitutes patient stabilisation and delivery. Recent advances in obstetric care have seen the emergence of conservative management prior to 32 weeks gestation.

Important issues that should be considered are:

1. Maternal evaluation
2. Fetal evaluation
3. Maternal monitoring
   - Invasive hemodynamic monitoring
   - Intravenous fluid management
   - Radiological monitoring
4. Fetal monitoring
5. Specific drug therapy

Some rapid acting antihypertensive agents are:

1. Dihydralazine
2. Labetalol
3. Nifedipine
4. Sodium nitroprusside

Drugs being evaluated for use as acute-acting antihypertensive agents are:

1. Isradipine
2. Nimodipine
3. Nicardipine
4. Nitrendipine
5. Ketanserin
6. Urapidil

Labetalol

Labetalol is an agent which confers antagonist activity directed at both alpha and beta adrenoreceptors. It is 4–8 times more effective in the case of beta than alpha adrenoreceptors. It produces its antihypertensive effect without compromising the maternal cardiovascular system by producing peripheral vasodilatation. This may help to maintain renal and uterine blood flow. Intravenous labetalol administered at 0.5 to 2 mg/kg produces an almost immediate fall in blood pressure with a minimal increase or decrease in heart rate. It is usually administered as a concomitant infusion which is initiated at 20 mg/hour. This may be increased by 20 mg increments every 10–20 minutes until appropriate blood pressure control is achieved, or a maximum total dose of 300 mg is administered.

Feto-placental blood flow remains unaltered with the use of labetalol.

Sodium nitroprusside

The fetomaternal adverse effects associated with sodium nitroprusside include fetal cyanide poisoning, transient fetal bradycardia, fetal metabolic acidosis and maternal hypotension.

Diazoxide

Diazoxide is a potent arteriolar vasodilator. In pregnant women it is administered as a 300 mg bolus injection. An important maternal adverse effect is severe precipitous hypotension. The adverse fetomaternal hemodynamic consequences of diazoxide administration can be improved by slow infusion of the drug. Diazoxide usage ought to be restricted to scenarios where the patient is unresponsive to dihydralazine, labetalol or nifedipine.

Nimodipine

Nimodipine is a calcium channel antagonist. It stabilises calcium channels, resulting in a calcium blockade. The drug is selectively effective on cerebral vasculature. Intravenous (15–45 μg/kg infusion) or sublingual administration (0.3 mg/kg) results in a decrease in blood pressure. Belforte et al have demonstrated a reduction in pulsatility index in maternal ophthalmic and central retinal arteries as well as reduction in systolic/diastolic ratios in the fetal middle cerebral arteries. The associated decrease in cerebral vasospasm is used to advantage in the treatment of patients with severe preeclampsia and eclampsia.

Conclusion

In a hypertensive crisis the main aims of therapy are to prevent cerebrovascular complications and to avoid progression of chronic hypertension into superimposed preeclampsia, which has a worse prognosis. The following factors need to be considered when choosing an appropriate antihypertensive agent:

- Effectiveness and safety
- Familiarity and experience with the agent
- Knowledge of doses and drug interactions
- Lack of maternal and fetal adverse effects
- Maintenance of uteroplacental blood flow
- Rapid onset of action
- Ease of administration of the drug

After initial treatment with a rapid acting agent it is recommended that oral therapy be introduced to maintain control of arterial blood pressure. Although delivery of the fetus is usually the definitive management of severe hypertension in pregnancy it should be appropriately timed and planned.

Currently, there is no ideal acute-acting antihypertensive for the pregnant patient. Dihydralazine, nifedipine and labetalol appear to be the most commonly used and recommended agents. Although there are many other rapid acting antihypertensive agents, they need to be subjected to large randomised controlled trials to assess the safety and efficacy. Until, then it is important that clinicians familiarise themselves with the drug they choose to use.

PRACTICE POINTS

- Preeclampsia causes significant morbidity and mortality. Maternal morbidity and mortality is partly related to cerebrovascular accidents. It is important to differentiate hypertensive urgencies from hypertensive emergencies. The pregnant patient with a systolic pressure over 169 mmHg or a diastolic blood pressure over 109 mmHg requires prompt, but gradual, reduction of high blood pressure.

- It is recommended that diastolic blood pressure not be reduced by more than 30 mmHg, and neither should the mean arterial pressure be reduced by more than 25 per cent.
- Appropriate fetomaternal evaluation is important prior to instituting antihypertensive therapy. Intravenous dihydralazine remains the most widely used rapid-acting antihypertensive agent as it is easy to administer, efficacious, inexpensive and most clinicians are familiar with its use.
- Recent studies suggest that nifedipine be considered the agent of choice in hypertensive emergencies. Labetalol is particularly useful in the scenario of ventricular tachycardia, or if dihydralazine fails to lower raised blood pressure. The use of sodium nitroprusside and diazoxide should be reserved for specific situations. Ketanserin and urapidil are newer agents; initial studies suggest that they have a potential role as rapid-acting antihypertensive agents.

Appendix 2. Cervical score

In induction of labour, success depends on the nature of the cervix (cervical score) and the method of induction.

Cervical scoring system

Score	0	1	2	3
Dilatation	Closed	1-2	3-4	>5
Length (cm)	>4	3-4	1-2	<1
Consistency	Firm	Average	Soft	
Position	Posterior	mid	Anterior	
Station of head	-3	-2	0	+1

Cervical score:

Favourable: 6 or more
Unfavourable: 5 or less

Methods of induction:

1. Stripping the membranes and amniotomy
2. Oxytocin drip 2.5 u in 500 ml of normal saline. Start with 20 drops a minute (5 miu/ml; each ml 20 drops; 5 miu/min) and increase by 10 drops every 20 min till 3 to 4 contractions occur in every 10 min (each lasting for 40 seconds). Drip is then maintained at that rate till delivery or 8 hours (if progress is good continue) or fetal distress.
3. Prostaglandins
   a. PGE_2 gel: Endocervical 0.2 mg; repeat 8 hours later if no response.
   b. Vaginal PGE_2: 3 mg pessary or 2–3 mg of gel.

c. PGE_1 or misoprostol 25 mg oral at 6 hour intervals; 2 doses as effective as 2 mg of vaginal PGE_2 (Dinoprostone) gel 2 insertions at 6 hours; almost two-thirds in each group delivered in 24 hours.

Vaginal 25 mg misoprostol 4 hourly 4 doses could be used safely for induction of labour. It is contraindicated in scarred uteri.

4. Foley's catheter has been used as an alternative method but it is contraindicated if there is history of vaginal bleeding, infection or rupture of membranes.

Index

OTHER TITLES FROM ORIENT LONGMAN

S.No.	Title	Author	Price (rupees)
1.	Clinical Gynecology (fourth edition)	K Bhasker Rao	235/-
2.	Clinical Methods in Obstetrics and Gynecology — A problem based approach	Edited by Asha Oumachigui et al	195/-
3.	Essential Management of Obstetric Emergencies	Thomas F Baskett	225/-
4.	Obstetrics and Gynecology for Postgraduates (second edition)	Edited by SS Ratnam et al Vol I Vol II	 550/- 600/-
5.	Practical Neonatal Care	Lalitha Krishnan	295/-
6.	Management of Labour	Edited by Arulkumaran S et al	300/-
7.	Urinary Incontinence	Edited by Vasan SS	570/-
8.	Gynecological Urology	Edited by Usha Saraiya and Shyam Deasi	250/-
9.	Low Birth Weight Baby	Edited by Tambyraja RL and Mongelli M	250/-
10.	Obstetric Medicine	Edited by Raman S and Chia P	200/-
11.	Perinatal Asphyxia	Edited by Arulkumaran S and Jenkins H	275/-